Fast Facts

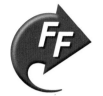

Fast Facts:
Epilepsy

Fifth edition

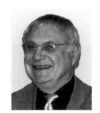

Martin J Brodie MB ChB MRCP MD FRCP
Director, Epilepsy Unit
Professor of Medicine and Clinical Pharmacology
Acute Services Division, Western Infirmary
Glasgow, Scotland, UK

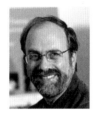

Steven C Schachter MS MD FAAN
Chief Academic Officer
Center for Integration of Medicine and Innovative
Technology
Professor of Neurology, Harvard Medical School
Boston, Massachusetts, USA

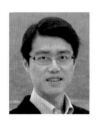

Patrick Kwan MB BChir FRCP PhD
Chair of Neurology
Department of Medicine
The University of Melbourne (RMH/WH)
Head of Epilepsy, Department of Neurology
Royal Melbourne Hospital
Parkville, Victoria, Australia

WITHDRAWN

Declaration of Independence
This book is as balanced and as practical as we can make it.
Ideas for improvement are always welcome: feedback@fastfacts.com

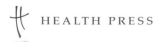

HEALTH PRESS

Fast Facts: Epilepsy
First published 1999; second edition 2001; third edition 2005; fourth edition 2009;
reprinted with revisions 2010, 2011
Fifth edition March 2012

Health Press Limited, Elizabeth House, Queen Street, Abingdon,
Oxford OX14 3LN, UK
Tel: +44 (0)1235 523233
Fax: +44 (0)1235 523238

Book orders can be placed by telephone or via the website.
For regional distributors or to order via the website, please go to:
fastfacts.com
For telephone orders, please call +44 (0)1752 202301 (UK, Europe and
Asia–Pacific), 1 800 247 6553 (USA, toll free) or +1 419 281 1802 (Americas).

Fast Facts is a trademark of Health Press Limited.

The authors wish to thank NC Sin MD, Hospital Authority Head Office, Hong
Kong, for supplying Figure 3.4 (which is also reproduced on the cover), Shih Hui
Lim MD, National Neuroscience Institute, Singapore, for supplying Figure 3.2 and
Howard L Weiner MD, Division of Pediatric Neurosurgery, New York University
Medical Center, New York, USA, for supplying Figures 6.1, 6.2 and 6.3.

The publisher and the authors have made every effort to ensure the accuracy of this
book, but cannot accept responsibility for any errors or omissions.

For all drugs, please consult the product labeling approved in your country for
prescribing information.

Registered names, trademarks, etc. used in this book, even when not marked as
such, are not to be considered unprotected by law.

A CIP record for this title is available from the British Library.

ISBN 978-1-908541-12-3

Brodie MJ (Martin)
Fast Facts: Epilepsy/
Martin J Brodie, Steven C Schachter, Patrick Kwan
Medical illustrations by Annamaria Dutto, Withernsea, UK.
Typesetting and page layout by Zed, Oxford, UK.
Printed by Latimer Trend & Company Limited, Plymouth, UK.

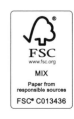

Text printed on biodegradable and recyclable paper
manufactured using elemental chlorine free (ECF) wood pulp
from well-managed forests.

FSC
www.fsc.org
MIX
Paper from
responsible sources
FSC® C013436

Abbreviations

ACTH: adrenocorticotropic hormone

AED: antiepileptic drug

CBZ: carbamazepine

CLB: clobazam

CNS: central nervous system

CT: computed tomography

CYP: cytochrome P450

CZP: clonazepam

DBS: deep brain stimulation

DEXA: dual-energy X-ray absorptiometry

EEG: electroencephalogram

ESL: eslicarbazepine acetate

ESM: ethosuximide

FBM: felbamate

FDA: Food and Drug Administration (USA)

fMRI: functional magnetic resonance imaging

GABA: gamma-aminobutyric acid

GBP: gabapentin

GTCS: generalized tonic–clonic seizure

JME: juvenile myoclonic epilepsy

LCM: lacosamide

LEV: levetiracetam

LTG: lamotrigine

MRI: magnetic resonance imaging

NTZ: nitrazepam

OXC: oxcarbazepine

PB: phenobarbital

PGB: pregabalin

PHT: phenytoin

PRM: primidone

RFN: rufinamide

RTG (EZG): retigabine (ezogabine)

SE: status epilepticus

SPECT: single photon emission computed tomography

SSRI: selective serotonin reuptake inhibitor

STP: stiripentol

SUDEP: sudden unexpected death in epilepsy

TCA: tricyclic antidepressant

TGB: tiagabine

TPM: topiramate

VGB: vigabatrin

VNS: vagus nerve stimulation

VPA: sodium valproate

ZNS: zonisamide

Glossary

Cryptogenic epilepsy: epilepsy presumed to have an underlying anatomic cause that remains unidentified

Cytochrome P450: a family of isoenzymes responsible for the hepatic oxidation of a range of lipid-soluble drugs

Dravet syndrome: a severe myoclonic form of epilepsy that begins in infancy

Enzyme inducer: a drug that increases synthesis of drug-metabolizing enzymes

Epilepsy: a chronic disorder of the brain characterized by an enduring disposition toward recurrent unprovoked seizures

Epilepsy syndrome: a constellation of characteristic seizures, abnormalities on EEG and/or brain imaging, response to therapy, prognosis, and associated clinical history and/or examination findings

Epileptogenesis: a sequence of events that converts a normal neuronal network into a hyperexcitable one resulting in the development of epilepsy

Generalized seizures: seizures that initially involve both hemispheres, usually with impairment of consciousness at the outset

Half-life (of drug): time taken for the plasma concentration of a drug to drop by 50%

Hypsarrhythmia: EEG pattern associated with infantile spasms, characterized by diffuse high-voltage spike-and-slow wave complexes, superimposed on a disorganized slow background

Idiopathic epilepsy: epilepsy that has a probable genetic basis

Incidence: the proportion of people developing a condition (new cases) in a given population within a specified time period

Ictal: relating to, or caused by, a seizure

Lennox–Gastaut syndrome: an encephalopathic syndrome that begins in early childhood involving multiple seizure types, major abnormalities on EEG and, usually, mental retardation

Localization-related epilepsy: epilepsy with partial-onset seizures (also called focal epilepsy)

Non-epileptic seizure event: an event that mimics a seizure without any identifiable neurophysiological abnormality (also called a pseudoseizure or psychogenic seizure)

Partial seizure: seizure arising from a particular part of the brain with ('complex partial') or without ('simple partial') impairment of consciousness

Pharmacogenomics: the study of the genetic determinants of drug response

Prevalence: the proportion of people in a given population with a diagnosed condition at any time

Seizure: transient symptoms and/or signs due to abnormal excessive or synchronous activity of a population of cortical neurons

Status epilepticus: continued or repeated seizure activity

Steady state (of drug): the inter-dosage range of serum concentrations achieved when the rate of administration equals the rate of elimination; occurs after approximately five elimination half-lives

Stevens–Johnson syndrome: severe idiosyncratic reaction to an antiepileptic drug characterized by skin eruption and mucosal and endothelial damage

Symptomatic epilepsy: epilepsy with an identified underlying cause

West syndrome: a rare condition characterized by the triad of infantile spasms, a typical hypsarrhythmic EEG pattern and arrest of psychomotor development

Introduction

Epilepsy – derived from the Greek word *epilambanein*, meaning 'to seize' or 'to attack' – was first recorded in the West as part of a Babylonian cuneiform treatise, known as 'Sakikku' or 'all diseases' on tablets dating from 716 BC to 612 BC, discovered in southern Turkey in 1951–2. The disorder was recognized around the same time in classical Chinese medical texts written from 770 to 221 BC. Hippocrates described epilepsy around 400 BC as 'the sacred disease', but most cultures placed a demonic interpretation on its unique constellation of symptoms and signs. It was only in 1875 that the English neurologist John Hughlings Jackson recognized a seizure as being due to disordered brain electricity.

Epilepsy is the most common serious neurological disorder in the world. Although this distressing condition remits in some people, many will have seizures throughout their lives. It affects all ages and crosses all geographic boundaries. Indeed, the commonest time to develop epilepsy in high-income countries is in old age, whereas in the developing world babies and young children are most often affected as a consequence of obstetric complications or neonatal infections.

The first edition of *Fast Facts: Epilepsy* was published in 1999 with information on seven second-generation antiepileptic drugs (AEDs). This was shortly after felbamate was reported to cause fatal aplastic anemia and hepatotoxicity, vigabatrin was shown to produce concentric visual field defects in 40% of exposed patients, and neurologists were becoming aware of the devastating complication of sudden unexpected death in epilepsy (SUDEP). At that time neurologists had not fully appreciated that seizures were often part of a spectrum of brain dysfunction, including cognitive, psychiatric and behavioral disorders. These problems can present not just during but also before the onset of epilepsy and require investigation and treatment in parallel to the management of seizures.

So what has been achieved in the past decade? Probably the most encouraging advances relate to the increasing range of imaging techniques, which open a window on the brain and provide fascinating insights into the function and dysfunction of this amazing piece of biotechnology. In parallel, the increasing precision of brain MRI offers the option of curative surgery to a wider range of people with drug-resistant focal epilepsy. The next 'big thing' could be the development of implantable devices aimed at interfering with epileptogenic or seizure-related processes in the brain, including systems that trigger the administration of therapy in response to sensing the electrical signals that produce the seizures. A device that delivers scheduled electrical stimulation bilaterally to the anterior nucleus of the thalamus has recently been approved in Europe and recommended for approval by the US Food and Drug Administration Devices Panel.

In 2012, the number of second-generation AEDs has risen to 15, with a few more to come over the next year or two. Whether their introduction has made a major contribution to outcomes for the catastrophic syndromes of infancy or the common adult epilepsies is under debate, but they do provide a wider range of options for both doctor and patient.

The other major area of optimism is that of genome analysis and the hope that it will provide insights into the causes of the individual epilepsy syndromes and help to target appropriate treatment. Clues are emerging that genetic markers can identify those patients likely to develop severe skin reactions with carbamazepine and the other AEDs so that their administration can be avoided in individuals at risk. Whether this area of research will also help to identify the best pharmacological choices for individual patients with epilepsy remains to be proven, but is highly likely.

In addition to incorporating the latest developments described above, we have updated all ten chapters in this fifth edition of *Fast Facts: Epilepsy*. We hope that this handbook will continue to be regarded as a succinct, practical and up-to-date aid for the busy clinician to help diagnose, investigate and successfully treat children and adults with a wide range of seizure disorders.

Incidence and prevalence

Epilepsy is the most common serious neurological condition. It affects nearly 70 million people in the world. In high-income countries, approximately 6 per 1000 people will develop epilepsy during their lifetime, and 45 people per 100 000 will develop new-onset epilepsy each year. These figures are nearly twice as high in low- and middle-income countries, possibly as a consequence of more primitive obstetric services as well as the greater likelihood of cerebral infection and head trauma.

Incidence varies greatly with age, with high rates in early childhood, low levels in early adult life and a second peak in people aged over 65 years (Figure 1.1). In recent years, there has been a fall in the number of children affected as well as a sharp rise in epilepsy in the elderly. Indeed, old age has now become the most common time in life to develop the condition.

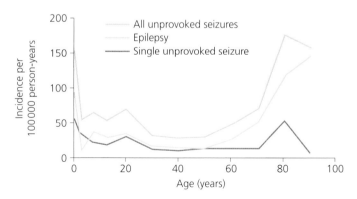

Figure 1.1 Incidence of single unprovoked seizures, epilepsy and all unprovoked seizures in Iceland between December 1995 and February 1999. Age-specific incidence of all unprovoked seizures was highest in the first year of life (130 per 100 000 person-years) and in those over 65 years old (110.5 per 100 000 person-years). Reproduced from Olafsson et al. © 2005, with permission from Elsevier.

Prognosis

Most patients with epilepsy have a good prognosis. The prognosis is strongly influenced by the underlying cause. In many people – particularly children – the condition will remit, although a substantial proportion will have epilepsy all their lives. Overall, 60–70% of patients become seizure free after the start of treatment with antiepileptic drugs (AEDs). Some of these patients become and remain seizure free on the initiation of the first AED, while in others the disorder appears to follow a more fluctuating course. Some patients can remain in remission after subsequent drug withdrawal, implying that the epileptogenic causes have truly remitted. The other 30–40% of patients continue to have seizures with varying degrees of frequency and severity. It is also increasingly recognized that some patients can have a 'remitting–relapsing' course, fluctuating between periods of seizure freedom and recurrence. Factors that indicate a poor prognosis for seizure control include:

- poor response to the initial AED treatment
- symptomatic cause
- high seizure frequency before AED treatment
- generalized tonic–clonic seizures
- generalized epileptiform activity on the electroencephalogram (EEG)
- family history of epilepsy
- comorbid psychiatric history.

Mortality

The standardized mortality ratio (the ratio of observed deaths to expected deaths) for patients with epilepsy is two to three times above that of the general population. In many cases, the cause of death is related to the underlying etiology, but sudden unexpected death in epilepsy (SUDEP) is believed to account for up to 17% of all epilepsy-related deaths. SUDEP has been defined as 'sudden, unexpected, witnessed or unwitnessed, non-traumatic and non-drowning death in patients with epilepsy, with or without evidence of a seizure, and excluding documented status epilepticus, in which postmortem examination does not reveal toxicological or anatomic cause of death'. The reported incidence of SUDEP ranges from 0.35 to 10 per 1000 patients per year. It is higher if the seizure disorder remains uncontrolled, suggesting that the majority of SUDEP is related to seizure activity. Other associated causes of death include drowning, burns, aspiration, pneumonia, status epilepticus and suicide.

Key points – epidemiology and prognosis

- Epilepsy is the most common serious neurological disorder.
- The incidence of epilepsy is highest in the elderly.
- Epilepsy can be controlled by antiepileptic drugs in the majority of patients.
- In general, a person with epilepsy is two to three times more likely to have an untimely death than someone in the general population.

Key references

Brodie MJ, Barry SJE, Bamagous GA et al. Patterns of treatment response in newly diagnosed epilepsy. *Neurology* 2012; in press.

Brodie MJ, Elder AT, Kwan P. Epilepsy in later life. *Lancet Neurol* 2009;8:1019–30.

Duncan S, Brodie MJ. Sudden unexpected death in epilepsy. *Epilepsy Behav* 2011;21:344–51.

Hitiris N, Mohanraj R, Norrie J et al. Predictors of pharmacoresistant epilepsy. *Epilepsy Res* 2007;75: 192–6.

Kwan P, Brodie MJ. Early identification of refractory epilepsy. *N Engl J Med* 2000;342:314–19.

Mohanraj R, Norrie J, Stephen LJ et al. Mortality in adults with newly diagnosed and chronic epilepsy: a retrospective comparative study. *Lancet Neurol* 2006;5:481–7.

Nashef L. Sudden unexpected death in epilepsy: terminology and definitions. *Epilepsia* 1997; 38(suppl 11):S6–8.

Ngugi AK, Bottomley C, Kleinschmidt I et al. Estimation of the burden of active and life-time epilepsy: a meta-analytic approach. *Epilepsia* 2010;51:883–90.

Ngugi AK, Kariuki SM, Bottomley C et al. Incidence of epilepsy: a systematic review and meta-analysis. *Neurology* 2011;77:1005–12.

Olafsson E, Ludvigsson P, Gudmundsson G et al. Incidence of unprovoked seizures and epilepsy in Iceland and assessment of the epilepsy syndrome classification: a prospective study. *Lancet Neurol* 2005;4:627–34.

Seizure types

A seizure is a symptom and represents the clinical manifestation of an abnormal and excessive synchronized discharge of a set of cortical neurons in the brain. Establishing the type(s) of seizure experienced by the patient has important implications for:

- selection of antiepileptic drugs (AEDs)
- likelihood of an underlying cerebral lesion
- prognosis
- possible genetic transmission.

Depending on the pattern of neuronal involvement, the clinical features of a seizure consist of a wide range of sudden and transitory abnormal phenomena, which may include alterations of consciousness, or motor, sensory, autonomic or psychic events. The widely used electroclinical classification of seizures established nearly three decades ago by the International League Against Epilepsy (ILAE) is the most widely adopted scheme. This classification system, viewed by the ILAE as a work in progress, divides seizures into two major groups: partial and generalized (Table 2.1).

Partial (or focal) seizures originate in a focal region of the cortex (Figure 2.1). They can be subdivided into those that do not impair consciousness (simple partial) and those that do (complex partial), which is useful for identifying patients whose safety may be compromised by loss of consciousness from their seizures. Partial seizures can also be classified according to their clinical manifestations, such as focal motor, and can spread rapidly to other cortical areas through neuronal networks, resulting in secondary generalized tonic–clonic seizures (Figure 2.2).

Simple partial seizures. The symptoms and signs of simple partial seizures depend on the site of origin of the abnormal electrical discharge. For example, those arising from the motor cortex cause rhythmic movements of the contralateral face, arm or leg (formerly

TABLE 2.1

International classification of epileptic seizures*

Partial (focal) seizures (beginning locally)
- Simple partial (without impaired consciousness)
  - with motor symptoms
  - with somatosensory or special sensory symptoms
  - with autonomic symptoms
  - with psychic symptoms
- Complex partial (with impaired consciousness)
  - simple partial onset followed by impaired consciousness
  - impaired consciousness at onset
- Partial, evolving into secondary generalized seizures

Generalized seizures (convulsive or non-convulsive)
- Absence
  - typical
  - atypical
- Myoclonic
- Clonic
- Tonic
- Tonic–clonic
- Atonic
- Unclassified

*Adapted from Commission on Classification and Terminology of the International League Against Epilepsy, 1981.

called Jacksonian seizures). Seizures arising from sensory regions or areas responsible for emotions and memory may produce olfactory, visual or auditory hallucinations, feelings of déjà vu or jamais vu, or fear, panic or euphoria.

Complex partial seizures, previously called temporal lobe or psychomotor seizures, are the most common seizure type in adults with epilepsy. There may be a warning, called an aura (simple partial seizure), immediately preceding loss or reduction of awareness. Complex partial seizures typically last less than several minutes. During that time, patients may appear awake, but lose contact with their environment; they do not respond normally to instructions or

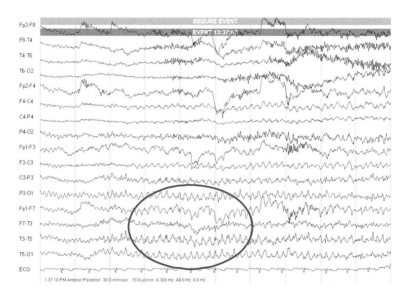

Figure 2.1 EEG showing a focal seizure over the left temporal area (circled).

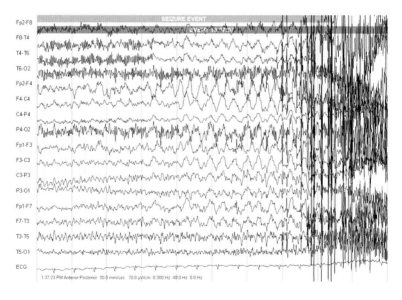

Figure 2.2 EEG showing secondary generalization from the partial-onset seizure in Figure 2.1.

questions during this time. Patients usually stare and either remain motionless or engage in repetitive semi-purposeful behavior called automatisms, including facial grimacing, gesturing, chewing, lip smacking, snapping fingers, repeating words or phrases, walking, running or even undressing. Patients cannot remember behaving in this manner. If restrained, they may become hostile or aggressive. After the seizure, patients are often sleepy and confused, and complain of a headache. This postictal state can last from minutes to hours.

Generalized seizures are characterized by widespread involvement of bilateral cortical regions at the outset and are usually accompanied by impairment of consciousness. The familiar tonic–clonic seizure (previously called 'grand mal') often starts with a cry. The patient suddenly falls to the ground and exhibits typical convulsive movements, sometimes with tongue or mouth biting and urinary incontinence.

Other subtypes of generalized seizures include absence, myoclonic, clonic, tonic and atonic seizures (see Table 2.1).

Absence seizures (previously called 'petit mal') mainly affect children.

Typical absence seizures usually last 5–10 seconds, commonly in clusters. They manifest as sudden onset of staring and impaired consciousness, with or without eye blinking and lip smacking. The electroencephalogram (EEG) typically shows a 3-Hz spike-and-wave pattern (Figure 2.3). There is a strong genetic component for the seizures as well as for the EEG abnormality. While absences will remit during adolescence in around 40% of patients, related tonic–clonic seizures may continue into adulthood.

Atypical absence seizures usually begin before 5 years of age in conjunction with other generalized seizure types and mental retardation. They last longer than typical absence seizures and are often associated with changes in muscle tone.

Myoclonic seizures consist of sudden brief muscle contractions, either singly or in clusters, that can affect any muscle group.

Clonic seizures are characterized by rhythmic or semi-rhythmic muscle contractions, typically involving the upper extremities, neck and face.

15

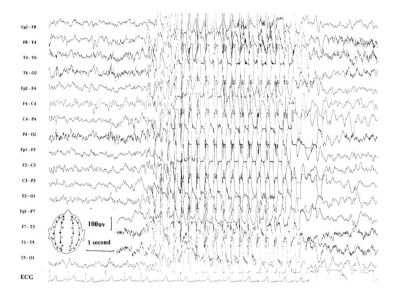

Figure 2.3 EEG showing the 3-Hz spike-and-wave pattern of a typical absence seizure, with characteristic abrupt onset and cessation.

Tonic seizures cause sudden stiffening of the extensor muscles, often associated with impaired consciousness and falling to the ground.

Atonic seizures (also called drop attacks) produce sudden loss of muscle tone with instantaneous collapse, often resulting in facial or other injuries.

Epilepsy syndromes

In addition to the classification of seizures, there is a separate system for epilepsies and epileptic syndromes (Table 2.2) that has been in place for many years. These are defined by groups of characteristic clinical features related to age at onset of seizures, family history of epilepsy, seizure type(s) and associated neurological symptoms and signs, aided by appropriate investigations, including EEG and brain imaging with, for example, CT and MRI (see Chapter 3, Diagnosis).

Diagnosing an epileptic syndrome helps the clinician define the likely prognosis, provide reasonable genetic counseling and choose the most appropriate AEDs.

TABLE 2.2

International classification of epilepsies and epileptic syndromes*

Localization-related (focal, local or partial)

- Idiopathic epilepsy with age-related onset
  - benign childhood epilepsy with centrotemporal spikes (benign rolandic epilepsy)
  - childhood epilepsy with occipital paroxysms
  - primary reading epilepsy
- Symptomatic epilepsy
- Cryptogenic epilepsy

Generalized

- Idiopathic epilepsy with age-related onset (listed in order of age at onset)
  - benign neonatal familial convulsions
  - benign neonatal non-familial convulsions
  - benign myoclonic epilepsy in infancy
  - childhood absence epilepsy
  - juvenile myoclonic epilepsy
  - epilepsy with generalized tonic–clonic seizures on awakening
  - other idiopathic epilepsies
- Cryptogenic or symptomatic epilepsy (listed in order of age at onset)
  - West syndrome (infantile spasms)
  - Lennox–Gastaut syndrome (childhood epileptic encephalopathy)
  - epilepsy with myoclonic–astatic seizures
  - epilepsy with myoclonic absence seizures
- Symptomatic epilepsy
  - non-specific syndromes (early myoclonic encephalopathy, early infantile epileptic encephalopathy)
  - specific syndromes (epileptic seizures as a complication of a disease, such as phenylketonuria, juvenile Gaucher's disease or Lundborg's progressive myoclonic epilepsy)

CONTINUED

17

TABLE 2.2 (CONTINUED)

Epilepsies undetermined whether focal or generalized

- With both generalized and focal features
  - neonatal seizures
  - severe myoclonic epilepsy in infancy
  - epilepsy with continuous spike waves during slow-wave sleep
  - acquired epileptic aphasia (Landau–Kleffner syndrome)
- Without unequivocal generalized or focal features[†]

Special syndromes

- Situation-related seizures
  - febrile convulsions
  - seizures related to other identifiable situations, such as stress, hormonal changes, drugs, alcohol withdrawal or sleep deprivation
- Isolated, apparently unprovoked epileptic events
- Epilepsies characterized by specific modes of seizure precipitation
- Chronic progressive epilepsia partialis continua of childhood

*Adapted from Commission on Classification and Terminology of the International League Against Epilepsy, 1989.
[†]Includes cases in which the clinical and EEG findings do not permit classification of the epilepsy as clearly generalized or localization-related, such as cases of tonic–clonic seizures during sleep.

Epileptic syndromes may be divided into:
- localization-related or focal epilepsies (those with partial-onset seizures)
- generalized epilepsies (those with generalized seizures).

Based on the knowledge of etiology, the syndromes are then further subdivided into:
- idiopathic – presumed to be genetic in origin
- symptomatic (secondary) – of known cause
- cryptogenic – presumed to be symptomatic but with an unidentified underlying abnormality.

The accuracy of classification depends on the extent of investigation.

With advances in technology, particularly in brain imaging, many subtle lesions can now be identified, making it possible to classify more of the epilepsies as symptomatic rather than cryptogenic. As with the classification of seizures, fueled by recent developments in diagnostic imaging and molecular genetics, the classification of epilepsy syndromes is also under revision by the ILAE.

Some of the epilepsy syndromes that may be encountered by the primary care provider are described below.

Benign rolandic epilepsy, also called benign childhood epilepsy with centrotemporal spikes, is an idiopathic focal epilepsy syndrome, with onset at 3–13 years of age. Nocturnal seizures predominate, and patients display a characteristic EEG pattern. Affected patients usually have normal cognitive function and normal findings on neurological examination. Seizures have a simple partial onset with occasional secondary generalization. Nocturnal seizures involve excessive salivation, gurgling or choking sounds, and clonic contractions of the mouth. Daytime seizures usually consist of tonic and/or clonic movements of one side of the body (particularly the face) and speech arrest, but the child remains conscious.

The EEG shows high-amplitude central and mid-temporal spikes and sharp waves, particularly during light sleep (Figure 2.4). The prognosis for children with benign rolandic epilepsy is excellent. The seizures are generally very easy to control with AEDs. The most commonly employed AEDs tend to be carbamazepine (CBZ), sodium valproate (VPA) and benzodiazepines given at bedtime. Other useful agents include oxcarbazepine (OXC) and levetiracetam (LEV). However, many children with mild or infrequent seizures do not require prophylactic AED treatment. Nearly all patients outgrow the disorder by their teenage years.

Juvenile myoclonic epilepsy (JME) is an under-recognized syndrome characterized by myoclonic jerks, tonic–clonic seizures or clonic–tonic–clonic seizures and, occasionally, absence seizures. Myoclonic seizures occur within the first few hours after arising from sleep (as

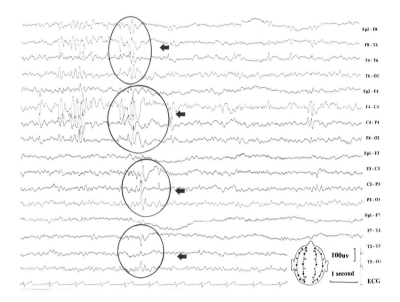

Figure 2.4 Interictal EEG of a patient with benign rolandic epilepsy showing mid-temporal (blue arrows) and central (red arrows) spikes and sharp waves.

do the generalized seizures), are mild and bilaterally symmetrical, and usually involve the upper extremities without impairing consciousness. The patient may spill or drop things during a myoclonic jerk. Less commonly, myoclonic seizures affecting the legs can cause falls.

JME is an inherited condition in otherwise neurologically normal children. It usually begins during the teenage years. The EEG shows a characteristic spike-and-wave pattern of 3.5–6 Hz, and multiple spike-and-wave complexes that may be precipitated by photic stimulation and sleep deprivation (Figure 2.5).

The AED of choice is VPA. Other useful drugs include lamotrigine (LTG), topiramate (TPM), zonisamide (ZNS) and LEV. Phenytoin (PHT), CBZ, OXC and gabapentin (GBP) may exacerbate the myoclonic seizures. The seizures respond well to treatment but usually recur when medication is withdrawn. Therefore, lifelong therapy is generally recommended.

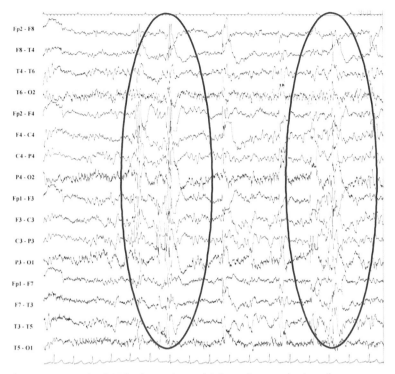

Figure 2.5 Interictal EEG of a patient with juvenile myoclonic epilepsy showing generalized, multiple spike-and-wave complexes (circled).

Febrile convulsions develop in association with fever (usually during the rapidly rising phase) with no evidence of another defined cause. They typically present between 6 months and 5 years old. There may be a family history of epilepsy. The incidence is approximately 4%. Up to 1 in 3 affected children will have recurrent febrile seizures. Although febrile seizures are generally benign, around 5% of children with febrile convulsions later develop epilepsy, typically in adolescence or later.

Factors associated with poor prognosis include seizures that have focal features or that last longer than 15 minutes, focal neurological abnormalities and a family history of afebrile seizures. Some children will go on to develop mesial temporal sclerosis and partial seizures that are often refractory to AED therapy.

Treatment of febrile convulsions is usually symptomatic, with sponge bathing and prompt administration of an antipyretic. Some physicians advocate prophylactic rectal diazepam when fever is present in children with a history of febrile convulsions. Most pediatric neurologists would not recommend long-term AED treatment for children with simple febrile seizures (i.e. generalized seizures lasting less than 15 minutes).

Infantile spasms are sudden brief seizures that are typically tonic flexor spasms of the waist, extremities and neck. They are usually seen as part of West syndrome, which is defined as infantile spasms, hypsarrhythmic patterns on the EEG and severe encephalopathy with psychomotor retardation. Infantile spasms are associated with 20% mortality; death usually results from the underlying pathology. Of the infants who survive, more than 75% are mentally retarded and more than 50% continue to have seizures throughout life.

Etiology may be known, for example cerebral malformations (half of all patients with tuberous sclerosis develop infantile spasms), perinatal brain damage and postnatal cerebral insults, or it may be idiopathic. Spasms typically begin before 12 months of age, with peak onset at 4–6 months. Seizures may occur dozens, if not hundreds, of times daily. In addition to massive flexor spasms, abduction or adduction of the arms, self-hugging movements and extensor contractions of the neck and trunk may be seen.

The EEG is markedly abnormal in most cases and consists of diffuse high-voltage spikes and slow waves superimposed on a disorganized slow background (hypsarrhythmia).

Infantile spasms are often difficult to control. Traditionally, adrenocorticotropic hormone (ACTH), corticosteroids, VPA and nitrazepam (NTZ) have been used. More recently, vigabatrin (VGB) has demonstrated superior efficacy to steroids and is now regarded as the treatment of choice by many pediatric neurologists for infantile spasms associated with tuberous sclerosis (see Chapter 5, Antiepileptic drugs).

Lennox–Gastaut syndrome is a devastating disorder beginning in childhood, which consists of mixed types of seizures and mental retardation. The EEG is characterized by slow (< 2.5 Hz) spike-and-wave patterns superimposed on an abnormal slow background.

Seizures typically occur daily, often in the tens or hundreds, and consist of axial tonic, tonic–clonic, atypical absence, myoclonic and atonic seizures, which often cause injuries. Brief tonic seizures usually occur during the night, sometimes in clusters. Atonic seizures may vary from head drops to catastrophic falls.

Cognitive deficit is usually present before the seizures develop and may be associated with behavioral problems. Most patients demonstrate abnormalities on neurological examination.

Prognosis for seizure remission is poor and response to AED therapy is generally unsatisfactory. Drugs showing some efficacy include VPA, LTG, TPM, clobazam (CLB), felbamate (FBM) and rufinamide (RFN).

Mesial temporal lobe epilepsy is a syndrome characterized by hippocampal sclerosis, which is the most common pathology in drug-resistant temporal lobe epilepsy. Onset of seizures usually occurs before puberty, often with a history of prolonged febrile convulsions in childhood. A seizure typically begins with vegetative auras, such as an epigastric rising sensation, or affective symptoms (most commonly fear), but may consist of complex delusional experiences, hallucinations, or olfactory or gustatory sensations. When the complex partial seizure ensues, impairment of consciousness is usually heralded by behavioral arrest and stare, followed by oro-alimentary, gestural and reactive automatisms lasting 1–2 minutes, which the patient does not remember. Afterwards, the patient is confused for varying periods. Postictal dysphasia may occur if the seizure involves the language-dominant hemisphere. Secondary generalization is relatively uncommon.

The diagnosis is supported by anterior temporal interictal spikes on a surface EEG, and hippocampal atrophy and signal change on MRI (Figure 2.6).

The disorder may initially respond well to AED treatment, but seizures often become drug resistant from early adulthood. However, if appropriately selected, up to 80% of patients with pharmacoresistant mesial temporal lobe epilepsy can be rendered seizure free by anterior temporal lobectomy.

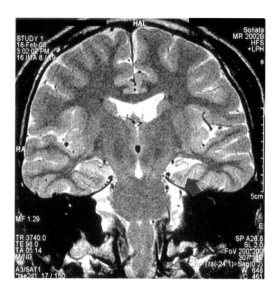

Figure 2.6 MRI scan of a patient with mesial temporal lobe epilepsy showing left hippocampal sclerosis (arrow).

Frontal lobe epilepsy. Frontal lobe seizures are the second most common type of seizures seen at epilepsy centers during presurgical evaluation for drug-resistant epilepsy. Because of the large size of the frontal lobe (40% of the entire cerebral cortex), a variety of clinical manifestations is seen in seizures arising from the different subregions. In general, frontal lobe seizures are shorter in duration than seizures arising from the temporal lobe, with a preponderance to cluster during nighttime. They have a strong motor component and consciousness is often preserved. Through involvement of the motor areas, there may be clonic movements of the extremities, trunk or face. Asymmetric tonic seizures are seen classically with tonic arm extension and elevation, and forced head deviation to the side of the extended arm, referred to as a fencing posture. In other forms, the seizures are described as 'hyperkinetic' with sudden and sometimes explosive onset of complex and violent behavioral automatisms. Patients may jump around, rotate or pound on objects, and commonly exhibit cycling or stepping movements. Motor features are often accompanied by vocalization, often in the form of a scream or grunts, though this vocalization can be part of understandable speech. Because of their often bizarre appearance, frontal lobe seizures are frequently misdiagnosed as psychogenic attacks.

Genetics

Epilepsy is part of the phenotype in more than 200 inherited disorders. Although numerous, genetic syndromes probably account for fewer than 1% of all cases of epilepsy. They often result in a developmental abnormality or an irreversible and progressive neuronal cell loss in the brain. Therefore, in these conditions, epilepsy is accompanied by other neurological deficits, such as learning disabilities, dementia or ataxia. Examples include a range of inherited metabolic disorders, mitochondrial encephalopathies and neuronal migration disorders.

A small number of inherited epilepsies are 'pure' idiopathic epilepsy syndromes, and there has been an explosion in our molecular understanding of these conditions over the past 15 years (Table 2.3).

TABLE 2.3

Examples of genes identified in inherited epilepsy syndromes

Syndrome	Gene	Gene product
Benign familial neonatal convulsions	KCNQ2 KCNQ3	Voltage-gated potassium channel subunits
Benign familial neonatal-infantile seizures	SCN2A	Voltage-gated sodium channel, α subunit, type 2
Autosomal-dominant nocturnal frontal lobe epilepsy	CHRNA4 CHRNB2 CHRNA2	Nicotinic acetylcholine receptor subunits
Autosomal-dominant lateral temporal lobe epilepsy	LGI1	Leucine-rich glioma-inactivated protein
Generalized epilepsy with febrile seizures plus (GEFS+)	SCN1A, SCN1B SCN2A GABRG2	Voltage-gated sodium channel subunits GABA$_A$ receptor, γ subunit, type 2
Severe myoclonic epilepsy of infancy	SCN1A	Voltage-gated sodium channel, α subunit, type 1

GABA, gamma-aminobutyric acid.

Key points – classification of seizures and syndromes

- A seizure is a symptom of brain dysfunction.
- Depending on the pattern of onset, seizures are broadly classified into partial (focal) and generalized types; classification is important for identifying the underlying cause, prognosis and best approach to management.
- Epileptic syndromes are defined by clinical features, aided by appropriate investigations that include EEG and brain imaging.
- Benign rolandic epilepsy occurs in otherwise neurologically normal children and generally has an excellent response to antiepileptic drugs (AEDs).
- Long-term AED treatment for children with simple febrile seizures is not recommended.
- Mesial temporal lobe epilepsy is often drug resistant but may be successfully treated by temporal lobectomy.
- Genetic mutations affecting ion channels have been identified in a range of rare idiopathic epilepsy syndromes.

Many genes have been identified, and the number is set to increase in the coming years.

In general, the presumptive causal mutations have been identified in large families with an autosomal-dominant inheritance pattern. Almost all mutations occur in genes that encode voltage-gated or ligand-gated ion channels. How these 'channelopathies' lead to recurrent episodic seizures remains unclear in most cases.

It has also become apparent that a specific mutation can give rise to a variety of phenotypes or clinical manifestations, and that a single seizure phenotype can be associated with different mutations.

It is important to point out that epilepsy syndromes with Mendelian inheritance are rare. The identification of mutations for these disorders provided initial target genes to be examined in the more common idiopathic epilepsy syndromes. That this 'candidate gene' approach has not yielded a significant discovery is probably a reflection of the complex inheritance and polygenic involvement in these common syndromes. Studies employing a more comprehensive approach to screen for a large number of variants covering the entire human genome (genome-wide association studies) are under way.

Identifying the genetic variants that predispose to the development of epilepsy can provide an insight into the mechanisms of excitability and seizure production, not only in genetically predetermined epilepsy but also in acquired types. It is also hoped that pharmacogenomics will provide a range of novel targets for future AED development.

Key references

Berg AT, Berkovic SF, Brodie MJ et al. Revised terminology and concepts for organization of seizures and epilepsies: report of the ILAE Commission on Classification and Terminology, 2005–2009. *Epilepsia* 2010;51:676–85.

Berg AT, Scheffer IE. New concepts in classification of the epilepsies: entering the 21st century. *Epilepsia* 2011;52:1058–62.

Camfield P, Camfield C. Epileptic syndromes in childhood: clinical features, outcomes, and treatment. *Epilepsia* 2002;43(suppl 3):27–32.

Commission on Classification and Terminology of the International League Against Epilepsy. Proposal for revised clinical and electroencephalographic classification of epileptic seizures. *Epilepsia* 1981;22:489–501.

Commission on Classification and Terminology of the International League Against Epilepsy. Proposal for revised classification of epilepsies and epileptic syndromes. *Epilepsia* 1989;30:389–99.

Helbig I, Scheffer IE, Mulley JC, Berkovic SF. Navigating the channels and beyond: unravelling the genetics of the epilepsies. *Lancet Neurol* 2008;7:231–45.

Nabbout R, Dulac O. Epileptic encephalopathies: a brief overview. *J Clin Neurophysiol* 2003;20:393–7.

Ng YT, Conroy JA, Drummond R et al. Randomized, phase III study results of clobazam in Lennox-Gastaut syndrome. *Neurology* 2011;77:1473–81.

Poduri A, Lowenstein D. Epilepsy genetics – past, present, and future. *Curr Opin Genet Dev* 2011;21: 325–32.

Reid CA, Berkovic SF, Petrou S. Mechanisms of inherited epilepsies. *Prog Neurobiol* 2009;87:41–57.

The diagnosis of epilepsy relies on the correct classification of epileptic seizures and epilepsy syndromes (see Chapter 2), with consequent implications for prognosis and choice of therapy.

Epilepsy is not a single disease but an extensive collection of conditions with a wide range of underlying etiologies and pathologies, all sharing the common and fundamental characteristic of recurrent, usually unprovoked, seizures. Figure 3.1 shows some common etiologies in relation to age.

The diagnostic procedure aims to answer three key questions.
- Is the episode an epileptic seizure?
- What is (are) the seizure type(s)?
- What is the epilepsy syndrome?

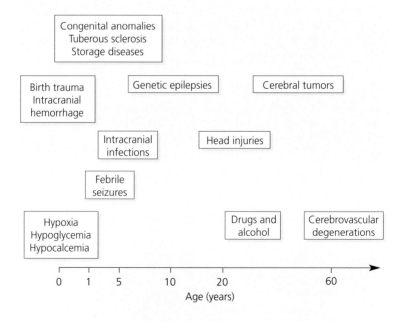

Figure 3.1 Etiology of epilepsy at different ages.

Differential diagnosis

A wide range of conditions can mimic epileptic seizures and must be considered in the differential diagnosis (Table 3.1). For example, syncopal attacks, sometimes with clonic movements and incontinence, are commonly misdiagnosed as epileptic seizures. Furthermore, non-epileptic psychogenic seizures (also called pseudoseizures) are estimated to occur in up to 45% of patients referred to specialist centers with apparently refractory epilepsy. This misidentification of non-epileptic conditions as epilepsy can lead to unnecessary treatments that are potentially harmful, and can delay the start of appropriate therapy. The temptation to attach a label of 'epilepsy' should be resisted if there is any doubt about the diagnosis despite a thorough evaluation. Both the physician and patient must simply await the passage of time before coming to a firm conclusion. Further challenges of diagnosis and management may arise in patients in whom non-

TABLE 3.1

Common differential diagnoses of seizures

Neurological	Endocrine/metabolic
• Transient ischemic attack	• Hypoglycemia
• Transient global amnesia	• Hyponatremia
• Migraine	• Hypocalcemia
• Narcolepsy	• Hypomagnesemia

Cardiac	Sleep disorders
• Vasovagal syncope	• Obstructive sleep apnea
• Reflex anoxic seizure	• Hypnic jerks
• Sick sinus syndrome	• Benign neonatal sleep myoclonus
• Arrhythmias	• REM sleep disorder
• Hypotension	

Psychological

• Non-epileptic psychogenic seizures

REM, rapid eye movement.

epileptic events coexist with epileptic seizures or develop as a substitute for epileptic seizures once the epilepsy is controlled.

Acute symptomatic seizures (also called provoked seizures) must be distinguished from unprovoked (epileptic) seizures. Acute symptomatic seizures occur in close temporal relationship (often arbitrarily defined as within 1 week) with an acute insult of the central nervous system (CNS), which may be metabolic, toxic, structural, traumatic, infectious or inflammatory. Common examples include seizures during an acute stroke, encephalitis or electrolyte disturbance. It has been estimated that up to 50% of all seizures may be considered to be acute symptomatic. There should be an adequate effort to search for any underlying acute CNS insult which may require urgent treatment. Unlike epileptic seizures, acute symptomatic seizures are not necessarily characterized by a tendency for recurrence. Therefore, as a general rule, long-term therapy with antiepileptic drugs (AEDs) is not indicated for most individuals, although it may be warranted on a short-term basis until the acute condition is resolved.

Clinical evaluation

Despite advances in investigational technologies, the diagnosis of epilepsy remains essentially clinical, and is based on a detailed description of the events experienced by the patient before, during and after a seizure. A witness's account of one or more of the episodes is an essential component of a confident diagnosis (Table 3.2). In addition to a full medical and social history, the patient should be asked about factors that may precipitate seizures by lowering the threshold for such an event (Table 3.3).

Physical examination is often unremarkable, although there may be focal neurological signs that correspond to an underlying structural abnormality in the brain. Investigations aiming to unearth anything that acutely provokes seizures should be guided by the clinical scenario. Routine blood tests should include full blood count and electrolytes, and an electrocardiogram should be performed to detect cardiac arrhythmias and conduction abnormalities, particularly prolonged QT syndromes. Drug screening may be carried out when the history suggests drug abuse. Lumbar puncture for cerebrospinal

TABLE 3.2

Important points to consider when taking a history from a patient suspected of having had one or more seizures

Features of the suspected seizure event

- Before the event
  - precipitating or provoking factors
  - preceding symptoms
  - duration of symptoms
- During the event
  - motor symptoms
  - sensory symptoms
  - level of awareness/ responsiveness
  - tongue biting or other injury
  - urinary incontinence
  - duration of event
- After the event
  - level of alertness
  - confusion
  - duration of symptoms
- Pattern of events
  - duration
  - frequency
  - stereotyped or variable

Patient's history

- Medical history
  - birth history
  - childhood febrile convulsion(s)
  - severe head trauma or other neurological insult
  - psychiatric illness
- Family history
- Drug history
  - prescribed medication
  - over-the-counter medication
  - illicit drugs
  - alcohol use

fluid examination should be reserved for those suspected of having an acute CNS infection.

Investigational technologies

Electroencephalography can support the clinical diagnosis of epilepsy and help with the classification of partial-onset or generalized seizures.

TABLE 3.3

Factors lowering seizure threshold

Common	Occasional
• Sleep deprivation	• Dehydration
• Alcohol withdrawal	• Barbiturate withdrawal
• Television flicker	• Benzodiazepine withdrawal
• Proconvulsive drugs	• Hyperventilation
• Systemic infection	• Flashing lights
• Head trauma	• Diet and missed meals
• Recreational drugs	• Specific 'reflex' triggers
• Non-compliance with antiepileptic drug therapy	• Stress
	• Intense exercise
• Menstruation	

It is important to give the electroencephalographer detailed information concerning the patient's age, seizure behavior and response to AEDs.

Routine EEGs are often insensitive – more than 50% of patients with epilepsy will have a normal trace. Activation techniques, including hyperventilation and photic stimulation (Figure 3.2), are helpful in uncovering abnormalities. Diagnostic yield can also be increased by repeat recordings. If the initial EEG is unremarkable and the diagnosis remains in doubt, a sleep-deprivation study is recommended.

Routine EEGs have a limited role in determining whether AED(s) can be safely tapered after a prolonged seizure-free interval. In a patient with suspected non-convulsive status epilepticus (see Chapter 7), an EEG can be diagnostic. An EEG can also immediately differentiate between epileptic and psychogenic convulsive status epilepticus.

Prolonged ambulatory recording. In cases of a negative routine EEG, better detection of interictal and ictal events may be achieved

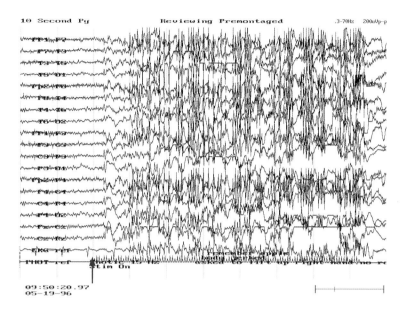

Figure 3.2 Photoconvulsive response provoked by intermittent photic stimulation. The arrow shows when photic stimulation began.

with a prolonged EEG recording using portable equipment. On the plus side, this allows recording to take place in the patient's usual environment, but technical faults are more likely and accurate correlation with simultaneous behaviors on video is available only with certain recording systems.

Video-EEG telemetry. Behavioral correlation can be achieved in inpatients by video monitoring during the EEG. This investigation is mandatory as part of the evaluation for epilepsy surgery, and may be the only way to distinguish epileptic from non-epileptic seizures.

Magnetoencephalography, in which the magnetic fields associated with the intracellular current flows within neurons are measured between seizures, has been the subject of recent research. In some situations, it usefully identifies candidates for surgery among patients with normal neuroimaging results.

EEG with functional MRI (fMRI). Recent advances in technology have allowed combined recording of EEG during fMRI, so that

33

interictal EEG changes can be spatially localized. As a result, simultaneous EEG and fMRI provides the opportunity to better understand the spatiotemporal mechanisms of the generation of epileptiform activity in the brain. Its role in the clinical management of epilepsy, particularly in selection of surgical candidacy in the case of drug resistance, is an area of active research.

Brain imaging

Structural imaging. Imaging studies of the brain to look for underlying structural abnormalities are essential for the appropriate diagnostic evaluation of most patients with epilepsy, particularly those presenting with partial-onset seizures. The imaging modality of choice is MRI. It has higher sensitivity and specificity than CT for identifying structural lesions such as malformations of cortical development (Figure 3.3a), hippocampal sclerosis, arteriovenous malformations, cavernous hemangioma (Figure 3.3b) and low-grade gliomas (Figure 3.3c). CT should be performed if MRI is unavailable and in patients for whom MRI is contraindicated (e.g. those with cardiac pacemakers, non-compatible aneurysm clips or severe claustrophobia).

Typical pathological findings vary with age. In children, MRI is particularly useful in identifying congenital abnormalities, such as neuronal migration disorders and arteriovenous malformations. In young adults, frequently detected conditions are hippocampal sclerosis, sequelae of head trauma, congenital anomalies, brain tumors and vascular lesions. For patients in mid-life and beyond, scans are helpful in evaluating stroke and cerebral degeneration, and in identifying primary and secondary neoplasia.

Any patient with refractory epilepsy in whom the initial MRI scan is normal should have a high-resolution scan to exclude hippocampal atrophy and focal cortical dysplasia. The scan should be repeated periodically if there is one of the following:

- suspicion of a tumor
- worsening in the patient's neurological or cognitive function
- increase in the frequency or severity of the seizures.

(a)

(b)

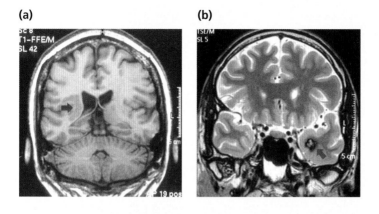

(c)

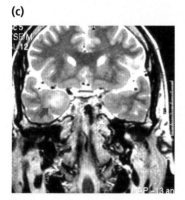

Figure 3.3 MRI scans showing (a) multiple gray matter heterotopia; (b) a cavernous hemangioma in the left temporal lobe; and (c) a low-grade glioma in the right temporal lobe.

Functional imaging can identify focal abnormalities in cerebral physiology even when structural imaging results are normal. Single photon emission computed tomography (SPECT) can demonstrate increased blood flow in brain regions in association with seizure activity. Epileptogenic areas can be detected as hypometabolic regions interictally by positron emission tomography (Figure 3.4). Magnetic resonance spectroscopy can measure changes in chemical compounds in the brain associated with neuronal loss in certain epileptogenic pathologies. Functional neuroimaging techniques have a limited role in routine diagnostic evaluation, but are useful adjuncts in the work-up for epilepsy surgery.

35

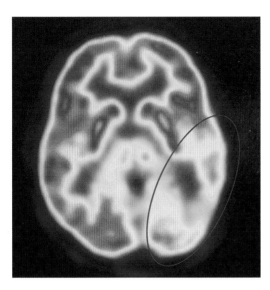

Figure 3.4 Positron emission tomography showing interictal hypometabolism over the left temporal and occipital areas (circled).

Key points – diagnosis

- Epilepsy has many underlying etiologies.
- A wide range of conditions can mimic epileptic seizures.
- A witness's account is essential for accurate diagnosis of epilepsy and classification of seizures.
- Electroencephalography can support diagnosis and help with the classification of seizures and syndromes.
- Structural brain imaging is essential in the diagnostic work-up for patients with seizures suspected of having a focal onset.
- MRI is the imaging modality of choice for detecting structural abnormalities in the brain.
- Functional neuroimaging techniques are mainly used as supplementary investigations in patients being considered for epilepsy surgery.

Key references

Binnie CD, Stefan H. Modern electroencephalography: its role in epilepsy management. *Clin Neurophysiol* 1999;110:1671–97.

Devinsky O, Gazzola D, LaFrance WC Jr. Differentiating between nonepileptic and epileptic seizures. *Nat Rev Neurol* 2011;7: 210–20.

Duncan JS. Imaging in the surgical treatment of epilepsy. *Nat Rev Neurol* 2010;6:537–50.

French JA, Pedley TA. Clinical practice. Initial management of epilepsy. *N Engl J Med* 2008; 359:166–76.

Krumholz A, Wiebe S, Gronseth G et al. Practice parameter: evaluating an apparent unprovoked first seizure in adults (an evidence-based review): report of the Quality Standards Subcommittee of the American Academy of Neurology and the American Epilepsy Society. *Neurology* 2007;69:1996–2007.

Scottish Intercollegiate Guidelines Network (SIGN). *Guideline No. 70 Diagnosis and Management of Epilepsy in Adults*. Edinburgh: SIGN, Royal College of Physicians, 2003. www.sign.ac.uk/guidelines/fulltext/70/index.html

Starting treatment

Several questions need to be addressed when deciding whether to prescribe an antiepileptic drug (AED) to a patient presenting after one or more seizures.

- What is the chance of recurrence?
- What are the potential negative consequences on the patient's life if seizures recur?
- What are the potential adverse effects of treatment?

After a single seizure. Whether treatment should be started after a single episode remains controversial. Depending on study methods and inclusion criteria, the probability of recurrence over the next 5 years after a single unprovoked seizure ranges from 31% to 71%. As a substantial proportion of such patients will not have further episodes, most specialists do not routinely recommend treatment after a single seizure. Prospective randomized studies have shown that, compared with delaying treatment until a further episode, immediate treatment after a first generalized tonic–clonic seizure (GTCS) does not improve the long-term remission rate. However, treatment should be considered after the first seizure when the chance of recurrence is high – for instance, in the presence of an underlying cerebral lesion, an abnormal EEG or a strong family history of epilepsy, or if the patient has an epilepsy syndrome such as juvenile myoclonic epilepsy (JME) that is characterized by a high likelihood of seizure recurrence. In some instances, the patient may wish to start treatment after a single event because they are concerned about the potentially significant impact that recurrent seizures could have on their lifestyle, such as their ability to legally drive a car.

After more than one seizure. Generally speaking, patients reporting more than one well-documented or witnessed seizure require treatment. Exceptions can include widely separated seizures,

provoked seizures for which specific treatments or avoidance
activity may be sufficient prophylaxis (e.g. concomitant illness
such as infection or metabolic disturbance, photosensitive epilepsy,
alcohol withdrawal) and certain benign childhood epilepsy
syndromes such as benign rolandic epilepsy (see page 19). In
addition, treatment is unlikely to succeed in patients unlikely or
unwilling to take medication as prescribed (e.g. some alcohol
abusers or drug addicts, or people who refuse to take medication
on principle).

An informed choice. The decision whether or not to start treatment
should be made after full discussion with the patient and their family
of the risks and benefits of both courses of action. The information
should be presented to the patient in the context of what is known and
what is conjecture about the risk of recurrent seizures, the chance of
a successful outcome with treatment and the likelihood of remission.
Pushing the issue if there is doubt about the diagnosis, particularly
if the patient resists the introduction of AED therapy, may be
counterproductive. Ideally, the patient and their immediate family
should be encouraged to make an informed commitment to the
treatment plan.

Reasons for taking prophylactic therapy should be discussed at the
outset. When prescribing an AED, the clinician must also discuss all
common side effects, as well as uncommon but serious drug-related
problems such as the risk of teratogenesis in women of childbearing
potential. That this particular risk has been touched upon should be
documented in the patient's case notes. Similarly, the regulations
regarding driving should be raised and documented. Time should be
taken to deal with the patient's fears, misconceptions and prejudices,
as well as those of the family. The importance of total compliance with
medication should also be stressed. These issues often require further
emphasis at subsequent visits. The possibility of sudden unexpected
death should be touched upon, especially if compliance is an issue or if
seizures remain uncontrolled (see page 10). The provision of written
material can be a useful way to ensure that nothing important has
been overlooked.

Principles of drug selection

The goal of treatment should be to enable the patient to lead as normal a lifestyle as possible, which generally requires complete seizure control without, or with minimal, side effects. Choosing the most suitable AED for an individual patient requires knowledge of the characteristics of the epilepsy, the patient and the available AEDs. The issues discussed below should be included in the decision-making process.

Monotherapy. In comparison with combination therapy, monotherapy is associated with better compliance and fewer side effects. It is therefore also likely to be more cost-effective. For these reasons, in general, serial monotherapy trials of two AEDs that are appropriate first-line treatment for the patient's seizure type(s) should be undertaken before combinations are tried (Figure 4.1). The chance of remission is highest with the first drug – 60% of patients with newly

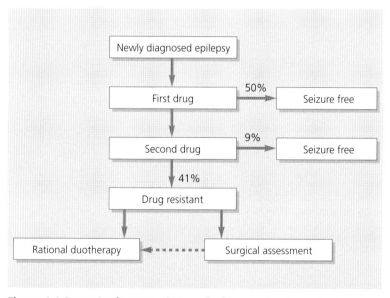

Figure 4.1 Strategies for managing newly diagnosed epilepsy. As shown, 59% of patients with newly diagnosed epilepsy achieve seizure control with the first or second drug, while 41% have drug-resistant epilepsy. Data from Brodie et al. 2012 (In press).

diagnosed epilepsy achieve seizure control with the first or second
AED. Substantial attention should therefore be given to choosing the
most appropriate initial AED, taking into account a range of factors,
including the seizure type(s) and/or epilepsy syndrome. Other relevant
issues include age, sex, weight, psychiatric and other comorbidities,
childbearing potential and concomitant medication.

Efficacy and tolerability. AED effectiveness is a function of efficacy
and tolerability. Given that lifelong treatment is often required, even in
patients with mild epilepsy, safety and lack of long-term sequelae are
also important considerations in addition to effectiveness when
selecting treatment.

Titration and monitoring. Approximately 50% of newly diagnosed
patients will be able to tolerate and become seizure free with the first
AED, often in low or moderate doses. In general, the AED should be
started at a low dose, with increments over a number of weeks to
establish an effective and tolerable regimen, although some agents,
such as sodium valproate (VPA) and levetiracetam (LEV), can be
commenced at effective doses with, or even without, a rapid titration
phase. Slow titration will help avoid concentration-dependent side
effects as with carbamazepine (CBZ) or topiramate (TPM), in
particular central nervous system toxicity, the presence of which is
likely to discourage the patient from persevering with therapy in the
long term. An additional benefit of a cautious approach is that it
allows the development of tolerance to sedation or cognitive
impairment. Such a policy will also ensure early detection of
potentially serious idiosyncratic reactions, such as rash, hepatotoxicity
and blood dyscrasias (see Side effects, pages 43–9). Slow titration with
lamotrigine (LTG) has been shown to reduce the risk of skin rash.

Measuring serum AED concentrations can help to determine the
extent of compliance, assess side effects and establish the most
effective dose for a seizure-free patient. Serum AED concentrations
associated with optimal control or with neurotoxicity vary from
patient to patient and may occur below, within or above the so-called
'therapeutic' or 'target' ranges for the drugs, particularly in children
and the elderly. These ranges should be regarded, therefore, purely as a

guide to prescribing. Routine measurement of serum levels of the newer AEDs is not otherwise recommended, as they do not correlate well on a population basis with efficacy or side effects.

Measurement of free serum phenytoin (PHT) concentrations can occasionally be useful when patients have low serum albumin levels or take other medications that bind tightly to protein. Women who experience an exacerbation of seizures just before their menses should have serum AED concentrations checked in the premenstrual period and compared with mid-cycle concentrations, as levels can drop markedly just before and during menstruation. This can be a particular problem with LTG.

If the first drug is well tolerated but the seizures persist, the dose should be increased towards the limit of tolerability, aiming for complete seizure freedom. If the first AED produces an idiosyncratic reaction or side effects at low or moderate doses, or fails to improve seizure control an alternative drug should be substituted.

Matching treatment to seizure type. The profile of activity against different seizure types differs among the AEDs (Tables 4.1 and 4.2). Certain epilepsy syndromes have been found to be particularly responsive to specific therapeutic agents. For instance, JME responds well to VPA, while many pediatricians regard vigabatrin (VGB) as the drug of choice for infantile spasms associated with tuberous sclerosis. On the other hand, myoclonic and absence seizures can be exacerbated by PHT, CBZ, gabapentin (GBP), pregabalin (PGB), oxcarbazepine (OXC), tiagabine (TGB) and eslicarbazepine acetate (ESL). It is therefore of paramount importance to classify the patient's seizure type(s) and epilepsy syndrome accurately (see Chapter 2). Recommended drug choices for adults and children according to seizure types are shown in Tables 4.3 and 4.4, respectively. The recommendations are based on the current literature and recent UK and US treatment guidelines. Because of the paucity of head-to-head comparative studies, particularly for the newer AEDs, the evidence base is supplemented by the authors' personal experience.

For partial seizures and GTCS (the most common seizure types), the established AEDs, with the exception of ethosuximide (ESM), appear to have similar efficacy. There is a possible small benefit of CBZ over

TABLE 4.1

Efficacy of established antiepileptic drugs against common seizure types and syndromes

Type of seizure/ syndrome	CBZ	CLB	CZP	ESM	PB	PHT	PRM	VPA
Partial	+	+	+	0	+	+	+	+
Secondary generalized	+	+	+	0	+	+	+	+
Tonic–clonic	+	+	+	0	+	+	+	+
Absence	–	?	?	+	0	–	0	+
Myoclonic	–	+	+	0	?+	–	?	+
Lennox– Gastaut	0	+	?+	0	?	0	?	+
Infantile spasms	0	?+	?+	0	?	0	?	+

+ proven efficacy; ?+ probable efficacy; 0 ineffective; – worsens control;
? unknown.
CBZ, carbamazepine; CLB, clobazam; CZP, clonazepam; ESM, ethosuximide;
PB, phenobarbital; PHT, phenytoin; PRM, primidone; VPA, sodium valproate.

VPA for partial seizures. Phenobarbital (PB) and primidone (PRM) have demonstrated higher withdrawal rates because of their sedative effects at higher dosages.

None of the newer AEDs has shown superior efficacy when tested against the established agents for the treatment of partial seizures and GTCS, but some have demonstrated better tolerability, in particular fewer neurotoxic side effects (Table 4.5). Thus, LTG and OXC have shown better overall effectiveness than CBZ and PHT, respectively, for partial epilepsy whereas VPA may be more efficacious than LTG for some generalized epilepsies.

Side effects. Safety concerns include idiosyncratic reactions, long-term complications and teratogenicity. The most common idiosyncratic reaction to AEDs is skin rash, which can range from a trivial evanescent exanthema (up to 5–10%) to rare but life-

TABLE 4.2

Efficacy of modern antiepileptic drugs against common seizure types and syndromes

Type of seizure/syndrome	ESL	FBM	GBP	LCM	LEV
Partial	+	+	+	+	+
Secondary generalized	+	+	+	+	+
Tonic–clonic	+	?+	?+	+	+
Absence	–	?+	–	?	?+
Myoclonic	–	?	–	?	+
Lennox–Gastaut	0	+	?	?	?
Infantile spasms	0	?	?	?	?

*Lamotrigine may worsen myoclonic seizures in some cases.
+ proven efficacy; ?+ probable efficacy; 0 ineffective; – worsens control;
? unknown.
ESL, eslicarbazepine acetate; FBM, felbamate; GBP, gabapentin; LCM, lacosamide;
LEV, levetiracetam; LTG, lamotrigine; OXC, oxcarbazepine; PGB, pregabalin; RFN,
rufinamide; RTG, retigabine (ezogabine in the USA); TGB, tiagabine;
TPM, topiramate; VGB, vigabatrin; ZNS, zonisamide.

threatening severe cutaneous reactions (Stevens–Johnson syndrome or toxic epidermal necrolysis), usually within 8 weeks of initiating treatment. Overwhelming evidence from recent studies found that carriers of the *HLA-B*1502* allele have a greatly increased risk of developing severe cutaneous reactions after taking CBZ. This allele is particularly prevalent (10–15%) in many Asian populations (including southern China, Taiwan, Thailand and Malaysia) but is rare (< 2%) in white populations. As a result of these findings, the US Food and Drug Administration (FDA), UK Medicines and Healthcare products Regulatory Agency (MHRA) and other national health regulators recommend testing for *HLA-B*1502* in individuals with ancestry from these areas before CBZ is initiated. The drug should be avoided if the patient is a carrier of this allele. Drug labeling has been amended by manufacturers accordingly. Until definitive evidence becomes available, clinicians should also consider avoiding the use of other AEDs associated with a high risk of severe cutaneous reactions (PHT,

LTG	OXC	PGB	RFN	RTG	TGB	TPM	VGB	ZNS
+	+	+	+	+	+	+	+	+
+	+	+	+	+	+	+	+	+
+	+	?	+	?	?	+	?+	+
+	−	−	+	−	−	?	−	?+
+*	−	−	?	−	?	+	−	+
+	0	?	+	0	?	+	?	?+
?+	0	?	?	0	?+	?+	+	?+

PB, LTG and OXC) in individuals known to have the allele. A similar association with *HLA-A*3101* has recently been reported in European and Japanese patients.

Felbamate (FBM) is associated with other idiosyncratic reactions including aplastic anemia and hepatotoxicity; as a consequence, it is relegated to the drug of last choice. Rare cases of acute glaucoma and clinically important hypohydrosis can complicate TPM administration; the latter has also been reported for zonisamide (ZNS).

Long-term use of some AEDs can lead to dysmorphic changes, such as gum hypertrophy with PHT, and weight gain with VPA, GBP and PGB. TPM and ZNS, on the other hand, often produce weight loss. VPA can also be associated with polycystic ovaries and hyperinsulinemia in susceptible women. The high incidence of concentric visual field defects in patients receiving VGB has substantially reduced the clinical use of this otherwise effective agent. Certain AEDs, such as PB, TPM, ZNS and VGB, are more commonly

TABLE 4.3

Choice of antiepileptic drugs in adolescents and adults according to seizure type*

Seizure type	First line	Second line/ add-on	Third line/ add-on
Absence (typical and atypical)	VPA ESM	LTG	LEV ZNS
Myoclonic	VPA	LEV ZNS TPM	LTG CLB CZP PB
Tonic–clonic	VPA CBZ LEV PHT PB[†]	LTG OXC	TPM ZNS PRM
Atonic	VPA	LTG TPM RFN	FBM
Simple and complex partial, with or without secondary generalization	CBZ PHT PB[†] OXC LTG TPM	VPA LEV ZNS GBP PGB LCM ESL RTG	TGB VGB FBM PRM
Unclassifiable	VPA LEV	LTG	TPM ZNS

*Other selection criteria include patient characteristics, side-effect profile, potential drug–drug interactions, availability and cost (see text).
[†]Phenobarbital is often regarded as second-line therapy because of sedation and behavioral problems.
CBZ, carbamazepine; CLB, clobazam; CZP, clonazepam; ESL, eslicarbazepine acetate; ESM, ethosuximide; FBM, felbamate; GBP, gabapentin; LCM, lacosamide; LEV, levetiracetam; LTG, lamotrigine; OXC, oxcarbazepine; PB, phenobarbital; PGB, pregabalin; PHT, phenytoin; PRM, primidone; RFN, rufinamide; RTG, retigabine (ezogabine in the USA); TGB, tiagabine; TPM, topiramate; VGB, vigabatrin; VPA, sodium valproate; ZNS, zonisamide.

TABLE 4.4

Choice of antiepileptic drugs in children according to seizure type*

Seizure type	First line	Second line/ add-on	Third line/ add-on
Absence (typical and atypical)	VPA ESM	LTG	CLB ZNS
Myoclonic	VPA LEV	TPM ZNS	LTG CLB PB
Tonic–clonic	VPA CBZ PB[†] LEV	LTG TPM PHT	ZNS OXC
Simple and complex partial, with or without secondary generalization	CBZ VPA LEV PB[†]	LTG TPM OXC ZNS	CLB PHT GBP[‡]
Infantile spasms	VGB ACTH	VPA NTZ	LTG ZNS TPM
Lennox–Gastaut	VPA	LTG TPM RFN	CLB FBM TPM
Unclassifiable	VPA LEV	LTG TPM	ZNS

*Other selection criteria include patient characteristics, side-effect profile, potential drug–drug interactions, availability and cost (see text).
†Phenobarbital is often regarded as second-line therapy because of sedation and behavioral problems. It is restricted for use in neonates in many developed countries.
‡Not approved for pediatric use.
ACTH, adrenocorticotropic hormone; CBZ, carbamazepine; CLB, clobazam; ESM, ethosuximide; FBM, felbamate; GBP, gabapentin; LEV, levetiracetam; LTG, lamotrigine; NTZ, nitrazepam; OXC, oxcarbazepine; PB, phenobarbital; PHT, phenytoin; RFN, rufinamide; TPM, topiramate; VGB, vigabatrin; VPA, sodium valproate; ZNS, zonisamide.

TABLE 4.5

Adverse effects of antiepileptic drugs on cognition and behavior

	Cognitive	Behavioral
Established AEDs		
Carbamazepine	+	0
Clobazam	+	+
Clonazepam	++	+
Ethosuximide	+	+
Phenobarbital	++	++
Phenytoin	+	0
Primidone	++	++
Sodium valproate	+	0
Modern AEDs		
Eslicarbazepine acetate	0	0
Felbamate	0	+
Gabapentin	0	0
Lacosamide	0	0
Lamotrigine	0	0
Levetiracetam	0	+
Oxcarbazepine	+?	0
Pregabalin	0	0
Retigabine†	0	0
Rufinamide	0	0
Tiagabine	0	0
Topiramate	+*	+
Vigabatrin	0	+
Zonisamide	0	+

*Risk reduced by slow titration.
†Ezogabine in the USA.
0 no effect; +? possible effect; + mild effect; ++ marked effect
AEDs, antiepileptic drugs..

associated with neuropsychiatric complications and should be used cautiously in patients with a history of mental illness. LEV can particularly produce emotional agitation and aggression.

The established AEDs have all been shown to increase the likelihood of fetal malformation. Recent analysis of several large-scale prospective registries suggests that the risk of major congenital malformation may be particularly high with VPA and perhaps also with PB compared with other established agents. Dose-dependent risk of major malformations has recently been associated with VPA, CBZ, PB and LTG administration. An association with facial clefts has been reported with TPM. Data regarding the newer AEDs are accumulating, and the teratogenic risk associated with LEV appears to be lower than with CBZ. Cognitive impairment may occur in children who were exposed to VPA in utero.

Pharmacokinetics and drug–drug interactions. An ideal AED should demonstrate complete absorption, linear kinetics and a long elimination half-life, allowing once- or twice-daily dosing. Low protein binding, lack of active metabolites and clearance by the renal route can also be regarded as advantageous, as a drug with these characteristics is likely to be easy to use and less likely to be implicated in pharmacokinetic interactions. However, the dose for drugs that are excreted unchanged by the kidney, such as GBP and PGB, will need to be adjusted in patients with renal impairment in relation to creatinine clearance.

Older AEDs are notorious for their ability to produce pharmacokinetic interactions among themselves as well as with other medications via their effect on the hepatic cytochrome P450 (CYP) enzyme system (Table 4.6). PB, PRM, PHT and CBZ induce CYP enzymes that accelerate the breakdown of many commonly prescribed lipid-soluble drugs metabolized by the same system, including oral contraceptives, cytotoxics, antiretrovirals, cardiac antiarrhythmics, immunosuppressants and warfarin. VPA is a weak CYP enzyme inhibitor, and as such can slow the clearance of other AEDs such as PHT and LTG. AEDs can also be targets for drugs other than AEDs that induce or inhibit hepatic metabolism. The newer AEDs are less

TABLE 4.6

Pharmacokinetic characteristics of antiepileptic drugs

	Undergoes hepatic metabolism	Affects drug-metabolizing enzymes	Associated with AED interactions
Established AEDs			
Carbamazepine	Yes	Yes	Yes
Clobazam	Yes	No	Yes
Clonazepam	Yes	No	Yes
Ethosuximide	Yes	No	Yes
Phenobarbital	Yes	Yes	Yes
Phenytoin	Yes	Yes	Yes
Primidone	Yes	Yes	Yes
Sodium valproate	Yes	Yes	Yes
Modern AEDs			
Eslicarbazepine acetate	Yes	Yes	Yes
Felbamate	Yes	Yes	Yes
Gabapentin	No	No	No
Lacosamide	Yes	No	No
Lamotrigine	Yes	No	Yes
Levetiracetam	No	No	No
Oxcarbazepine	Yes	Yes	Yes
Pregabalin	No	No	No
Retigabine*	Yes	No	Yes
Rufinamide	Yes	Yes	Yes
Tiagabine	Yes	No	Yes
Topiramate	Yes	Yes	Yes
Vigabatrin	No	No	Yes
Zonisamide	Yes	No	Yes

*Ezogabine in the USA. AEDs, antiepileptic drugs.

likely to interfere with hepatic metabolism, although OXC, FBM, rufinamide (RFN) and ESL, and TPM at daily doses above 200 mg, selectively induce the breakdown of the estrogenic component of the oral contraceptive pill.

Comorbidities. As well as controlling seizures, some AEDs have demonstrated efficacy for the treatment of other conditions that may coexist with epilepsy (Table 4.7). For instance, VPA has traditionally been used in bipolar affective disorder. It is also effective prophylaxis for migraine, an indication for which TPM has also been approved. GBP is effective for the treatment of certain neuropathic pain syndromes, while PGB has demonstrated efficacy for neuropathic pain and generalized anxiety disorder. LTG has recently been licensed for bipolar disorder. With a widening spectrum of indications, AED selection may be tailored according to the patient's neurological and psychiatric comorbidities (see Chapter 9, Quality of life).

TABLE 4.7
Antiepileptic drugs with efficacy in non-epileptic conditions*

Neuropathic pain
Carbamazepine
Oxcarbazepine
Lamotrigine
Gabapentin
Pregabalin
Lacosamide

Migraine prophylaxis
Sodium valproate
Topiramate

Essential tremor
Primidone
Topiramate

Anxiety
Gabapentin
Pregabalin
Clobazam

Bipolar disorder
Carbamazepine
Oxcarbazepine
Valproate
Lamotrigine

*Indications for non-epileptic conditions vary among different countries.

Bone health. Long-term AED therapy can lead to hypocalcemia and decrease biologically active vitamin D levels, resulting in reduced bone mineral density and higher risk of fractures. Most of the available data pertain to the older drugs, but information regarding newer agents is emerging. Both enzyme-inducing and non-enzyme-inducing agents are implicated, and the effects may be additive. A variety of mechanisms for AED-induced osteoporosis have been suggested, the most important of which appears to be an increased rate of bone turnover. Bone loss can be detected by dual-energy X-ray absorptiometry (DEXA) or quantitative ultrasound.

To reduce the risk of osteoporosis, patients taking long-term AED therapy are advised to maintain the optimal level of physical activity, a balanced diet and exposure to sunshine. They should be advised against smoking and excessive intake of alcohol or caffeine, all of which can exacerbate bone loss. Risk factors for osteoporosis include:
• prolonged AED therapy
• exposure to multiple drugs
• a non-ambulatory lifestyle
• concomitant corticosteroid therapy.
People at risk are advised to take calcium and vitamin D supplements and undergo regular DEXA scans. Once osteopenia or osteoporosis has developed, the patient should be referred to an endocrinologist for appropriate therapy (see *Fast Facts: Osteoporosis*).

Suicidality. Late in 2008, the FDA announced it would require warnings concerning suicidal thoughts or behavior in the prescribing information for all AEDs based on its meta-analysis of a large number of controlled clinical trials involving the newer AEDs. The FDA's announcement put the increased risk in perspective, saying that it amounted to one additional case of suicidal thoughts or behavior for every 500 patients treated with AEDs compared with placebo. As more data become available, comorbid depression is increasingly being implicated as a causative factor rather than the AEDs themselves. Nonetheless, clinicians should monitor patients closely for suicidal ideation when starting or increasing doses of AEDs.

Combination therapy can be considered if two successive monotherapy attempts with first-line AEDs are ineffective, as the chance of successful seizure control with a third choice of monotherapy is slim. If the first AED produces a good response but complete seizure freedom remains elusive, adding a drug with a different mechanism of action may be a more pragmatic strategy than substitution for some patients. Combination therapy reduces seizure frequency or severity in some patients.

The number of possible two-drug regimens is growing rapidly. Some evidence supports the suggestion that combinations involving a sodium channel blocker and a drug that facilitates the inhibition of gamma-aminobutyric acid (GABA) or a drug with multiple mechanisms of action are particularly beneficial. The only combination, however, for which there is hard evidence of synergism is that of VPA and LTG. Some useful combinations are listed in Table 4.8.

The practical difficulty with combination therapy is that troublesome or disabling side effects are common at high doses, and complex pharmacokinetic interactions can occur. Consequently, it is

TABLE 4.8

Useful antiepileptic drug combinations

Combination	Indication
Sodium valproate and ethosuximide	Generalized absences
Carbamazepine and sodium valproate	Complex partial seizures
Sodium valproate and lamotrigine*	Partial/generalized seizures
Topiramate and lamotrigine	Partial/generalized seizures
Vigabatrin[†] and lamotrigine	Partial seizures
Vigabatrin[†] and tiagabine	Partial seizures

*This is the only combination for which good laboratory and clinical evidence exists in support of synergism.
[†]Because of the high incidence of concentric visual field defects, vigabatrin should be reserved for patients in whom other antiepileptic drugs have failed or for infantile spasms secondary to tuberous sclerosis.

TABLE 4.9

Ten commandments in the pharmacological treatment of epilepsy

- Choose the correct drug for the seizure type and/or epilepsy syndrome
- Start at a low dose unless the patient is having frequent seizures
- Titrate up slowly to allow the development of tolerance to CNS side effects
- Keep the regimen simple with once- or twice-daily dosing, if possible
- Measure drug concentration to monitor compliance and to correlate with later seizure control and side effects
- Counsel the patient early regarding the implications of the diagnosis, the prophylactic nature of drug therapy, the importance of perfect compliance and the risk of SUDEP
- Try two reasonable AEDs as monotherapy before adding a second drug in combination
- When seizures persist, combine the best-tolerated first-line drug with one of the newer agents depending on seizure type and mechanisms of action
- Simplify medication schedules and regimens as much as possible in patients receiving polypharmacy
- Aim for the best seizure control consistent with optimal quality of life in patients with drug-resistant epilepsy

AED, antiepileptic drug; CNS, central nervous system; SUDEP, sudden unexpected death in epilepsy.

advisable to combine drugs with different side-effect profiles and those that do not have the potential for deleterious drug interactions. Practical guidelines for prescribing AEDs are summarized in Table 4.9.

Drug-resistant epilepsy

The International League Against Epilepsy (ILAE) defines drug-resistant epilepsy as 'a failure of adequate trials of two tolerated and appropriately chosen and used AED schedules (whether as monotherapies or in combination) to achieve sustained seizure freedom'. Fulfillment of the definition in a patient should prompt a comprehensive review of the diagnosis and management, preferably by an epilepsy specialist.

Work-up for epilepsy surgery can be considered at this point, particularly if a potentially operable structural abnormality, such as mesial temporal sclerosis, has been identified. This is also a good time to evaluate whether there may be any factor responsible for a state of 'pseudoresistance' (Table 4.10), by reviewing:

- security of the diagnosis
- accuracy of the seizure and/or syndrome classification
- results of brain imaging
- compliance with medication

TABLE 4.10

Some reasons for 'pseudoresistance' to antiepileptic drug therapy

Wrong diagnosis

- Syncope, cardiac arrhythmia, for example
- Malingering, psychogenic non-epileptic seizures
- Underlying brain neoplasm

Wrong drug(s)

- Inappropriate for seizure type
- Pharmacokinetic/pharmacodynamic drug interactions

Wrong dose

- Too low (if target range is ignored)
- Side effects preventing dose increase

Wrong lifestyle

- Poor compliance with medication
- Inappropriate choices (e.g. alcohol or drug abuse)

- the presence of negative lifestyle factors, such as erratic sleeping habits or covert alcohol or drug abuse.

If the first AED combination is ineffective and epilepsy surgery is not an option, a sequence of drug combinations with potential complementary modes of action could be tried. Data to guide further pharmacological management are lacking. A small proportion of patients will become seizure free with three AEDs, but treatment with four or more is highly unlikely to be tolerated and therefore successful. Drug burden is a function of dose as well as number of drugs, and so further introductions may be made possible by reducing the dose of one or more AEDs.

Therapy withdrawal

Successful treatment outcome can be regarded as freedom from seizures without side effects. Individuals in whom treatment is successful are more likely to lead rewarding lives – with optimal intellectual and emotional development, and positive educational and vocational achievements – than patients with uncontrolled, particularly daytime, seizures. In short, they will have a better chance of fulfilling their potential. Eventually, many patients can have their medication withdrawn and remain in remission.

Patients who are 'doing well' may want to stop treatment for a variety of reasons, including the awareness of side effects or the subjective perception of subtle deterioration in cognitive function. Some patients do not equate taking medication with normal health. Finally, the patient may want to start a family and may be concerned about the possible negative effects of AEDs on reproductive function, along with the specter of teratogenesis.

Several studies have shown that after a long period of perfect seizure control, medication can be stopped without seizure recurrence (for several years at least) in around 60% of patients. There are no data to guide the length of the seizure-free period. In children, 2 years of seizure freedom is reasonable before considering AED withdrawal. Although there is no defined timescale, a flexible 5-year seizure-free period would be more prudent in adults.

Seizure type or epilepsy syndrome is not absolutely predictive of recurrence. However, a few specific childhood syndromes, such as benign rolandic epilepsy and benign familial neonatal convulsions, tend to do well after drug withdrawal, whereas JME has a high probability of relapse. Some forms of idiopathic generalized seizures, either absence or tonic–clonic, are less likely to recur once they are under control. Even complex partial seizures can disappear after a long period of freedom from seizures.

The highest probability of remaining seizure free can be seen in patients with the following characteristics:

- relatively few seizures before and after starting AED therapy
- treatment with a single AED
- seizure free for many years
- normal neurological examination
- no structural lesion on brain imaging.

The EEG is not a huge help in predicting seizure recurrence, but a normal investigation is reassuring.

There are no standard protocols defining optimal regimens for tapering medication. Most specialists advise slow reduction by increments over at least 6 months. If the patient is taking two AEDs, one drug should be slowly withdrawn before the second is tapered. More than 90% of recurrences will occur during the year following withdrawal, and many will present during or shortly after the tapering period.

Referral to a specialist

The primary goal of epilepsy management is to restore the patient's functional capacity to its maximal potential. Attaining this goal is often a team effort involving medical and social service professionals and the patient's family, friends and coworkers. The role of the primary care provider varies according to the clinical setting, their experience and the patient's needs.

Primary care physicians must be familiar with all the diagnostic and therapeutic options, because they will usually perform the initial evaluation of the first seizure, primarily to exclude non-epileptic causes such as syncope and hypoglycemia. Even experienced doctors may not feel qualified, however, to assume full responsibility for the diagnosis, planning and follow-up of patients with epilepsy. Often, they do not have direct access to the necessary investigational techniques. If a non-epileptic cause of the symptoms is ruled out, the patient should see a neurologist or other appropriate specialist for further diagnostic studies to determine the likelihood of further seizures and to consider the need for, and choice of, AED therapy.

Dose adjustments can be undertaken later by the primary care physician. The patient should be referred back to the epilepsy specialist if:

- seizures are unresponsive to the first two AED schedules
- treatment causes significant side effects
- a pregnancy is being planned
- he or she is considering stopping therapy.

Attending to the patient's psychosocial, cognitive, educational and vocational needs is an important part of caring for people with epilepsy. Both the primary care physician and the epilepsy specialist should work closely with other medical and social service professionals, and extend their roles beyond that of clinician to educator and advocate. Subsequent referral to a comprehensive epilepsy center for EEG monitoring, investigational drugs or devices, or consideration for epilepsy surgery is indicated for compliant patients whose seizures prove resistant to two or three reasonable attempts at pharmacological manipulation using new and established AEDs singly and in combination.

Key points – pharmacological management

- Patients reporting more than one unprovoked seizure usually require treatment; treatment after a single unprovoked seizure could be considered if the chance of recurrence is high.
- At the start of treatment, a single antiepileptic drug (AED) should be given at a low dose and slowly titrated to an effective dose.
- First-line AEDs should be chosen according to the patient's seizure type(s) and/or epilepsy syndrome. Other important factors include the likelihood of side effects, lack of long-term sequelae, and a low potential for pharmacokinetic interactions.
- Combination AED therapy could be used after failure of two monotherapies in series or if the first AED is well tolerated but fails to completely control the seizures.
- Drug-resistant epilepsy is defined as failure of adequate trials of two tolerated and appropriately chosen and used AED schedules (whether as monotherapies or in combination) to achieve sustained seizure freedom.
- A small number of patients will demonstrate a sustained response to the fourth, fifth, sixth or even seventh regimen, and so drug-resistant epilepsy should never be viewed nihilistically.
- None of the newer AEDs has shown superior efficacy when tested against established agents for the treatment of partial seizures and generalized tonic–clonic seizures, although some may be better tolerated.
- Patients should be referred to a specialist for definitive diagnosis and initiation of treatment, or when seizures prove refractory to medication, they are planning for pregnancy or hoping to stop treatment in the case of remission.
- The primary care physician should play an important role in coordinating professional care for people with epilepsy.

Key references

Brodie MJ, Barry SJE, Bamagous GA et al. Patterns of treatment response in newly diagnosed epilepsy. *Neurology*; 2012; in press.

Brodie MJ, Covanis A, Lerche H et al. Antiepileptic drug therapy: Does mechanism of action matter? *Epilepsy Behav* 2011; 21:331–41.

Brodie MJ, Elder AT, Kwan P. Epilepsy in later life. *Lancet Neurol* 2009;8:1019–30.

Brodie MJ, Holmes GL. Should all patients be told about sudden unexpected death in epilepsy (SUDEP)? Pros and cons. *Epilepsia* 2008;49(suppl 9):99–101.

Brodie MJ, Sills GJ. Combining antiepileptic drugs – rational polytherapy? *Seizure* 2011;20: 369–75.

Compston JE, Rosen CJ. *Fast Facts: Osteoporosis*, 6th edn. Oxford: Health Press, 2008.

Costa J, Faraleira F, Ascencau R et al. Clinical comparability of the new antiepileptic drugs in refractory partial epilepsy: a systematic review and meta-analysis. *Epilepsia* 2011; 52:1280–91.

Kaufman KR. Antiepileptic drugs in the treatment of psychiatric disorders. *Epilepsy Behav* 2011; 21:1–11.

Kwan P, Arzimanoglou A, Berg AT et al. Definition of drug resistant epilepsy. Consensus proposal by the ad hoc Task Force of the ILAE Commission on Therapeutic Strategies. *Epilepsia* 2010;51: 1069–77.

Kwan P, Schachter SC, Brodie MJ. Drug-resistant epilepsy. *N Engl J Med* 2011;365:919–26.

Loring DW, Marino S, Meador KJ. Neuropsychological and behavioural effects of antiepileptic drugs. *Neuropsychol Rev* 2007;17:413–25.

Man CBL, Kwan P, Baum L et al. Association between HLA-B*1502 allele and antiepileptic drug-induced cutaneous reactions in Han Chinese. *Epilepsia* 2007;48:1015–18. Erratum in *Epilepsia* 2008;49:941.

Marson AG, Al-Kharusi A, Alwaidh M et al. The SANAD study of effectiveness of carbamazepine, gabapentin, lamotrigine, oxcarbazepine, or topiramate for treatment of partial epilepsy: an unblinded randomised controlled trial. *Lancet* 2007;369:1000–15.

Marson AG, Al-Kharusi A, Alwaidh M et al. The SANAD study of effectiveness of valproate, lamotrigine, or topiramate for generalised and unclassifiable epilepsy: an unblinded randomised controlled trial. *Lancet* 2007;359: 1016–26.

Marson A, Jacoby A, Johnson A et al. Immediate versus deferred antiepileptic drug treatment for early epilepsy and single seizures: a randomised controlled trial. *Lancet* 2005;365:2007–13.

McCormack M, Alfirevic A, Bourgeois S. HLA-A*3101 and carbamazepine – induced hypersensitivity reactions in Europeans. *N Engl J Med* 2011; 364:1134–43.

Meador KJ, Baker GA, Browning N et al. Cognitive function at 3 years of age after fetal exposure to antiepileptic drugs. *N Engl J Med* 2009;360:1597–1605.

Patsalos PN, Berry DJ, Bourgeois BFD et al. Antiepileptic drugs – best practice guideline for therapeutic drug monitoring. *Epilepsia* 2008; 49:1239–76.

Perucca E. Clinically relevant drug interactions with antiepileptic drugs. *Br J Clin Pharmacol* 2005;61: 246–55.

Perucca E, Tomson T. The pharmacological treatment of epilepsy in adults. *Lancet Neurol* 2011;10:446–56.

Petty SJ, O'Brien TJ, Wark JD. Anti-epileptic medication and bone health. *Osteoporos Int* 2007;18: 129–42.

Stephen LJ, Brodie MJ. Selection of antiepileptic drugs in adults. *Neurol Clin* 2009;27:967–92.

Tomson T, Battino D, Bonizzoni E et al. Dose-dependent risk of malformations with antiepileptic drugs. An analysis of data from the EURAP epilepsy and pregnancy registry. *Lancet Neurol* 2011;10: 609–17.

Zaccara G, Franciotta D, Perucca E. Idiosyncratic adverse reactions to antiepileptic drugs. *Epilepsia* 2007;48:1223–44.

Established antiepileptic drugs

Despite the recent entry into the marketplace of a wide range of new pharmacological options, most patients still receive treatment with one of the older antiepileptic drugs (AEDs). Comparative pharmacokinetics, indications and a guide to dosing in children and adults are summarized in Tables 5.1–5.3.

Chapter 4 sets out the main principles of drug selection and overall pharmacological management. Here, the use of each drug is considered in terms of its mechanism of action, indication, dosage, tolerability, pharmacokinetics and drug–drug interactions. Problems likely to be encountered in everyday clinical practice are highlighted.

Carbamazepine (CBZ) was synthesized by Schindler at Geigy in 1953 in an attempt to compete with the newly introduced antipsychotic chlorpromazine. The first clinical studies in epilepsy were not carried out until 1963. CBZ acts by preventing repetitive firing of action potentials in depolarized neurons via use- and voltage-dependent blockade of sodium channels.

Indications. Over the years, CBZ has gained acceptance as a first-line treatment for partial and tonic–clonic seizures. It is not effective for, and may even exacerbate, generalized absences and myoclonic seizures.

Dosage. CBZ should be introduced at low doses (100–200 mg daily) with 100–200 mg increments every 3–14 days, depending on the urgency of the situation. Slow introduction facilitates tolerance to its central nervous system (CNS) side effects and allows hepatic auto-induction of CBZ metabolism to take place. The dose can be increased over the first month or two to a maintenance amount that completely controls the seizure disorder. A balance must be achieved in the individual patient between speed of seizure control and acceptance of temporary CNS toxicity. The final dose will depend on the extent to which CBZ induces its own metabolism (Figure 5.1).

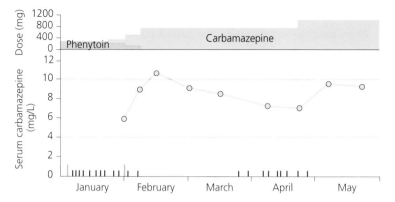

Figure 5.1 Auto-induction of carbamazepine metabolism. The lines at the bottom of the graph represent partial (pink) and tonic–clonic (green) seizures.

Despite this careful approach, some patients will be unable to tolerate the neurotoxic side effects of CBZ, even at low doses and serum concentrations. Diplopia, headache, dizziness, nausea and vomiting are the most common complaints. For some patients with drug-resistant epilepsy, these symptoms cause a dose ceiling, which may be less than an effective dose. High peak concentrations often result in intermittent side effects around 2 hours after dosing, necessitating administration three or four times daily in some patients. Such problems can be overcome by prescribing a controlled-release formulation that can be given twice daily, or by shifting a greater percentage of the total daily dose to bedtime, particularly when the patient has only nocturnal or early morning seizures.

Side effects. In addition to the CNS toxicity described above, CBZ can cause a range of idiosyncratic reactions, the most common of which is a morbilliform rash in 5–10% of patients (Figure 5.2). Other unusual, but more severe, skin eruptions include erythema multiforme and Stevens–Johnson syndrome. To minimize the risk of the latter, individuals with ancestry from broad areas of Asia should be tested for *HLA-B*1502* before CBZ is initiated. CBZ should be avoided if the patient tests positive (see Side effects, pages 43–5). Another allele, *HLA-A*3101*, has recently been identified in European and Japanese patients who develop

TABLE 5.1

Pharmacological properties of established antiepileptic drugs

Drug	Mode(s) of action	Indications (seizure type)	Absorption (bioavailability %)
Carbamazepine	Blocks fast-inactivated state of Na^+ channel	Partial, GTCS	Slow (75–80)
Clobazam	Activates $GABA_A$ receptor	Partial, generalized	Rapid (90–100)
Clonazepam	Activates $GABA_A$ receptor	Partial, generalized	Rapid (80–90)
Ethosuximide	Blocks low-voltage-activated Ca^{++} channel	Absence	Rapid (90–95)
Phenobarbital	Activates $GABA_A$ receptor	Partial, GTCS, myoclonic, tonic, clonic, SE	Slow (95–100)
Phenytoin	Blocks fast-inactivated state of Na^+ channel	Partial, GTCS, SE	Slow (85–90)
Primidone	Activates $GABA_A$ receptor	Partial, GTCS	Rapid (90–100)
Sodium valproate	Various actions on multiple targets	Partial, generalized	Rapid (100)

GABA, gamma-aminobutyric acid; GTCS, generalized tonic–clonic seizure; SE, status epilepticus.

a range of skin reactions with CBZ. Reversible mild leukopenia often occurs within the first few months of treatment, but therapy does not need to be discontinued unless there is also evidence of infection or if the white-cell count slips well below 2000×10^9/liter. Potentially fatal blood dyscrasias and toxic hepatitis are much rarer problems. At high

Protein binding (% bound)	Elimination half-life (hours)	Routes of elimination	Target serum concentration
70–80	24–45 (single) 8–24 (chronic)	Hepatic metabolism Active metabolite	4–12 mg/L (17–50 µmol/L)
87–90	10–30	Hepatic metabolism Active metabolite	None
80–90	17–56	Hepatic metabolism	None
0	20–60	Hepatic metabolism 25% excreted unchanged	40–100 mg/L (283–706 µmol/L)
48–54	72–144	Hepatic metabolism 25% excreted unchanged	10–40 mg/L (40–172 µmol/L)
90–93	9–40	Saturable hepatic metabolism	10–20 mg/L (40–80 µmol/L)
20–30	4–12	Hepatic metabolism Active metabolites 40% excreted unchanged	8–12 mg/L (25–50 µmol/L)
88–92	7–17	Hepatic metabolism Active metabolite	50–100 mg/L (350–700 µmol/L)

concentrations, the drug has an antidiuretic-hormone-like action that can result in fluid retention in elderly patients or in those with cardiac failure. Mild hyponatremia is usually asymptomatic, but if the serum sodium level falls below 120 mmol/liter the patient may present with confusion, peripheral edema and deterioration in seizure control. A dose-dependent

TABLE 5.2

Dosing guidelines for established antiepileptic drugs in adults

Drug	Starting dose (mg/day)	Commonest dose (mg/day)	Maintenance dose (mg/day)	Dosing interval
Carbamazepine	200	600	400–2000	bd–qds
Clobazam	10	20	10–40	od–bd
Clonazepam	1	4	2–8	od–bd
Ethosuximide	500	1000	500–2000	od–bd
Phenobarbital	60	120	60–240	od–bd
Phenytoin	200	300	100–700	od–bd
Primidone	125	500	250–1500	od–bd
Sodium valproate	500	1000	500–3000	bd–tds

od, once daily; bd, twice daily; tds, three times a day; qds, four times a day.

TABLE 5.3

Dosing guidelines for established antiepileptic drugs in children

Drug	Starting dose (mg/kg/day)	Maintenance dose (mg/kg/day)	Dosing interval
Carbamazepine	5	10–25	bd–qds
Clobazam	0.25	0.5–1	od–bd
Clonazepam	0.025	0.025–0.1	bd–tds
Ethosuximide	10	15–30	od–bd
Phenobarbital	4	4–8	od–bd
Phenytoin	5	5–15	od–bd
Primidone	10	20–30	od–bd
Sodium valproate	10	15–40	bd–tds

od, once daily; bd, twice daily; tds, three times a day; qds, four times a day.

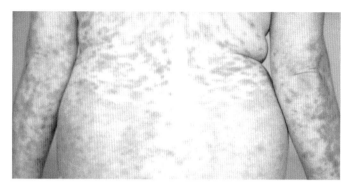

Figure 5.2 Typical morbilliform rash caused by carbamazepine.

increase in major malformations has been reported in children who were exposed to CBZ in utero.

Pharmacokinetics and drug–drug interactions. As well as inducing its own metabolism, CBZ can accelerate the hepatic breakdown of a number of lipid-soluble drugs. The most common interaction is with the oral contraceptive pill, necessitating a daily estrogen dose of 50 μg or more for most women. Other important interactions are with sodium valproate (VPA), ethosuximide (ESM), corticosteroids, anticoagulants, antipsychotics, cytotoxics, antiretrovirals, statins and immunosuppressants.

Drugs that inhibit CBZ metabolism resulting in toxicity include phenytoin (PHT), cimetidine, dextropropoxyphene, diltiazem, erythromycin, isoniazid, verapamil, viloxazine and fluoxetine. The substantial variation of CBZ concentrations in any given patient over the course of a day – as much as 100% with twice-daily dosing – makes the interpretation of concentration monitoring problematic unless the times of dosing and blood sampling are standardized. In many patients, the dose can be titrated adequately on clinical criteria alone. Exceptions include patients suspected of poor compliance and those taking a cocktail of AEDs that are likely to interact with one another.

Clobazam (CLB). The structure of CLB (1,5-benzodiazepine) differs slightly from those of clonazepam (CZP) and diazepam (1,4-benzodiazepines), which may account for the lower propensity of CLB to produce sedation.

Indications. CLB is a useful adjunctive drug for drug-resistant partial and generalized seizures. Recent studies have supported its efficacy for children with Lennox–Gastaut syndrome.

Dosage. Short-term administration (e.g. 20 mg daily for 3 days) can be an effective strategy in women with premenstrual seizure exacerbations and for other patients as 'cover' for holidays or stressful events, such as weddings and surgery. A single dose of 10–30 mg can have a useful prophylactic action if taken immediately after the first event in patients who regularly suffer clusters of complex partial and secondary generalized seizures. Children with Lennox–Gastaut syndrome should be given 0.5–2 mg/kg/day.

Not all responders will maintain a worthwhile improvement in seizure control on long-term dosing owing to the development of tolerance. Nevertheless, a substantial proportion (10–20%) of patients treated with CLB become seizure free. Intermittent use of CLB reduces the likelihood of tolerance.

Side effects. As already mentioned, CLB is less likely to cause sedation than the 1,4-benzodiazepines. Nevertheless, depression, irritability and tiredness have been reported. As with barbiturates, deterioration in behavior and mood disturbance can occur, particularly in patients with learning disabilities; CLB should probably be avoided in such patients.

Pharmacokinetics and drug–drug interactions. CLB is biotransformed in the liver to a number of metabolites, including an active metabolite N-desmethylclobazam. Comedication with enzyme-inducing AEDs increases the metabolism of CLB, and hence the N-desmethylclobazam level. The clinical relevance of this interaction has not been established.

Clonazepam (CZP), like other benzodiazepines, enhances inhibition mediated through gamma-aminobutyric acid (GABA).

Indications. CZP is primarily used as adjunctive treatment for generalized seizures such as absence, myoclonic and atonic seizures. It is also effective against partial and tonic–clonic seizures. Parenteral CZP can be used for status epilepticus.

Dosage. Adults should be started on 0.5–1.0 mg daily with subsequent weekly increments as necessary. In children, 0.5 mg daily is the usual starting dose. Tolerance to the anticonvulsant effect and difficulty weaning patients off CZP limit its clinical value.

Side effects are prominent, usually dose limiting, and include sedation, ataxia and behavioral changes, such as depression.

Pharmacokinetics and drug–drug interactions. Drug interactions of CZP are minimal, although its half-life in adults can be slightly reduced from 17–56 hours (as monotherapy) to 12–46 hours in the presence of an enzyme-inducing AED.

Ethosuximide (ESM) was introduced in 1958. It works by reducing T-type calcium currents in thalamic neurons.

Indications. Since its introduction, ESM has been the drug of choice for children with absence seizures who do not also have tonic–clonic or myoclonic seizures. ESM is also effective for atypical absences, but ineffective for myoclonic, tonic–clonic and partial-onset seizures.

Dosage. In children and adults, dosing is initiated with 500 mg daily (250 mg daily in children under 6 years of age), with 250-mg dose increments as clinically indicated over 2–3 weeks to the maximum tolerated amount, which is typically 15–30 mg/kg once or twice daily in children and 20–40 mg/kg given in two divided doses in adults. Serum concentrations less than 40 mg/liter are usually ineffective.

Side effects occur in approximately 40% of patients and predominantly relate to the gastrointestinal tract (hiccups, nausea, vomiting, abdominal pain, anorexia). Headache, dizziness, drowsiness and unsteadiness may also occur. Allergic rashes are seen in up to 5% of patients. A transient leukopenia has been described.

Pharmacokinetics and drug–drug interactions. The metabolism of ESM is hepatic, protein binding is minimal and drug interactions are not a major problem.

Phenobarbital (PB), synthesized in 1912, is the oldest AED in common clinical use. It enhances the effect of GABA by prolonging chloride channel opening at the $GABA_A$ receptor, resulting in neuronal hyperpolarization.

Indications. Once widely prescribed for partial and tonic–clonic seizures, PB has been relegated to second-line therapy in some countries because it causes sedation and behavioral problems. Nevertheless, the drug appears to be effective and well tolerated in experience from developing countries. Indeed, on a global scale PB remains one of the most important AEDs because of its low cost and continuing widespread use in the developing world and in many industrialized countries. The parenteral formulation is occasionally useful as adjunctive therapy in SE. PB may also be used for myoclonic seizures.

Dosage. In children, doses of 2–5 mg/kg daily are usually necessary for optimal seizure control. Resulting serum concentrations typically range from 15 to 40 mg/liter. Maintenance doses in adults range from 60 to 240 mg/day. Tapering should be attempted slowly (e.g. 15 mg/month) to minimize the possibility of withdrawal seizures and other undesirable symptoms, such as altered mood and sleep disturbance.

Side effects. As mentioned above, PB often causes sedation and behavioral problems, such as depression and agitation. In addition, it may cause hyperactivity in children and elderly patients. Recent data suggest an increased risk of fetal abnormalities in infants exposed to the drug during the first trimester of pregnancy. Other problems include allergic rash, osteoporosis, folate deficiency and Dupuytren's contracture.

Pharmacokinetics and drug–drug interactions. The half-life of PB is 4 days. Consequently, steady-state serum concentrations may not be reached for up to 3 weeks after a change in dose. PB is metabolized in the liver, and is a powerful inducer of hepatic metabolism, accelerating the clearance of many other lipid-soluble drugs.

Phenytoin (PHT). The discovery and clinical testing of PHT by Merritt and Putnam in the 1930s introduced both a major new non-sedating AED and an animal model of epilepsy (electrical seizures in the cat). Like CBZ, PHT blocks voltage-dependent neuronal sodium channels.

Indications. For the past 80 years, PHT has been a first-line medication for the prevention of partial and tonic–clonic seizures and for the acute treatment of seizures and SE, although it is more often used as a second-line agent in children. PHT is not effective against myoclonic, atonic and absence seizures. It is available in oral and intravenous forms.

Dosage. Depending on the urgency of the situation, PHT may be started at the maintenance dose, typically 300 mg daily as a single dose or in two divided doses in adults (5–8 mg/kg daily in children), or at a higher dose, such as 20 mg/kg divided into three oral doses over 24 hours or 20 mg/kg given intravenously – no faster than 50 mg/ minute. The dose should be increased at 1–2 weekly increments as necessary and as tolerated. Most adults usually achieve satisfactory seizure control with once-daily dosing. Patients with erratic compliance should be treated twice daily to lessen the effect of a missed dose.

Side effects can be divided into neurotoxic symptoms (ataxia, nystagmus, dysarthria, asterixis, somnolence) that typically present 8–12 hours after an oral dose, chronic dysmorphic effects (gingival hyperplasia, hirsutism, acne, facial coarsening) that occur after months of therapy, and uncommon long-term problems (folate deficiency, osteopenia, peripheral neuropathy, cerebellar atrophy) that take years to develop. PHT is associated with rash in approximately 5% of patients. Other rare idiosyncratic reactions include Stevens–Johnson syndrome, hepatitis, bone-marrow suppression, lymphadenopathy and a lupus-like syndrome. PHT may also be a teratogen.

Pharmacokinetics and drug–drug interactions. PHT is metabolized in the liver. The first step of this process involves the enzyme arene oxidase, which has saturable kinetics, particularly at moderate-to-high serum concentrations. The concentration at which PHT pharmacokinetics become non-linear varies as a function of age. As a consequence of this pharmacokinetic profile, small changes in dosing may result in disproportionate changes in serum concentration (Figure 5.3). In all patients, the dose should be increased or decreased in 25–50 mg increments when clinically indicated, particularly when serum concentrations exceed 10 mg/liter. Serum concentrations should then be checked after 1–2 weeks.

PHT induces hepatic enzymes and may, therefore, reduce serum concentrations of metabolized AEDs such as CBZ, VPA, lamotrigine

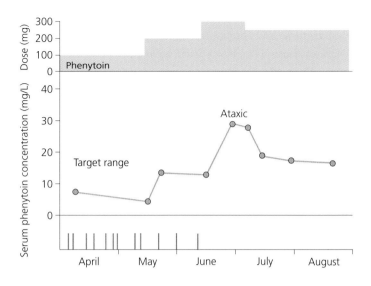

Figure 5.3 Saturation kinetics with phenytoin. The lines at the bottom of the graph represent occurrence of tonic–clonic seizures. Seizures in this illustrative case tended to occur in association with serum phenytoin concentrations below the mid-target range.

(LTG) and topiramate (TPM). The effectiveness of other lipid-soluble drugs, including oral contraceptives and anticoagulants, is also jeopardized. PHT is tightly bound to circulating albumin and may be displaced by other drugs; some of these, such as VPA, also inhibit the metabolism of PHT. Checking free PHT serum concentrations may be useful clinically to correlate with a patient's possible neurotoxic symptoms in the setting of hypoalbuminemia, renal and hepatic insufficiency, or pregnancy. Febrile illness may increase the clearance of PHT, resulting in lowered serum concentrations. Enteral feeding has been reported to decrease PHT absorption.

Fosphenytoin is a phosphate ester prodrug of PHT that can be administered intravenously or intramuscularly. It is water soluble and can be given more rapidly than intravenous PHT, with fewer local side effects. Although more expensive, fosphenytoin is better tolerated than parenteral PHT and may replace the latter in the standard treatment of SE (see Chapter 7).

Primidone (PRM) is metabolized in the liver to PB and another active substance, phenylethylmalonamide. It is not fully understood how much of a role the latter plays in the overall antiepileptic effect of PRM.

Indications. PRM is effective against partial and generalized tonic–clonic seizures, but appeared to be inferior to CBZ and PHT in clinical trials, largely because of its relatively poor tolerability (see below). Therefore, it is primarily used as adjunctive therapy.

Dosage. Dosing should be started with 125 mg at bedtime, increasing by 125 mg every 3–5 days as tolerated to 500–1500 mg daily in two or three divided doses. As with PB, discontinuation of PRM should be very gradual.

Side effects. PRM has a higher incidence of side effects than CBZ, PHT and PB, particularly sedation and ataxia. Decreased libido or impotence associated with PRM use has been reported.

Pharmacokinetics and drug–drug interactions. As its half-life is shorter than that of PB, concentrations of PB are usually higher than those of PRM. Like PB, PRM is a powerful enzyme inducer.

Sodium valproate (VPA). The anticonvulsant property of VPA was recognized serendipitously in 1963 when it was used by Pierre Eymard as a solvent for a number of other compounds. VPA exerts its antiepileptic property, at least in part, by limiting sustained repetitive firing by a use- and voltage-dependent effect on sodium channels. It also facilitates the effects of the inhibitory neurotransmitter GABA.

Indications. VPA is now established as effective over the complete range of seizure types, with particular value in the idiopathic generalized epilepsies.

Dosage. The starting dose for adults and adolescents should be 500 mg once or twice daily. Alterations thereafter can be made according to the clinical status of the patient. Divalproex sodium (a combination of valproic acid and VPA) can also be given twice daily. As the drug can take several weeks to become fully effective, frequent dose adjustments shortly after therapy is started may be unwarranted. Because VPA does not exhibit a clear-cut concentration–effect–toxicity relationship and daily variations in concentration at a given dose are

73

wide, routine monitoring is unhelpful unless closely correlated with the patient's clinical situation. A few patients need and tolerate serum concentrations up to 150 mg/liter.

Side effects. Unpleasant or distressing side effects include dose-related tremor, weight gain due to appetite stimulation, thinning or loss of hair (usually temporary) and menstrual irregularities including amenorrhea. Some young women develop polycystic ovary syndrome associated with obesity and hirsutism. Rarely, stupor and encephalopathy associated with hyperammonemia can occur. The insidious development of parkinsonism has also been reported, although this effect reverses on VPA withdrawal. Hepatotoxicity, histologically a microvesicular steatosis similar to that found in Reye's syndrome, affects fewer than 1 in 20 000 exposed individuals. This appears to be a particular concern in children under 3 years of age receiving AED polypharmacy, some of whom will have a coexistent metabolic defect. Other sporadic problems include thrombocytopenia and acute pancreatitis.

An important concern in women of childbearing potential is an increased dose-dependent risk of major malformations in offspring exposed to VPA during the first trimester of pregnancy. Recent data from prospective pregnancy registries suggest the risk may be more than 10%, including an estimated 1–3% risk of neural tube defects, at high dosage (> 1000 mg daily). Women of childbearing potential should not be started on VPA without specialist neurological advice. High-dose VPA has also been linked to cognitive impairment in children who were exposed to the drug in utero.

Pharmacokinetics and drug–drug interactions. VPA can inhibit a range of hepatic metabolic processes, including oxidation, conjugation and epoxidation reactions. Targets include other AEDs, particularly PHT, PB, the active epoxide metabolite of CBZ, and LTG. VPA does not, however, interfere with the hormonal components of the oral contraceptive pill.

Modern antiepileptic drugs
After a hiatus of nearly 20 years, 15 new AEDs and two devices – the vagus nerve stimulator and deep brain stimulator (see pages 103–6) – have received licenses for the adjunctive treatment of refractory

epilepsy, the last so far only in Europe. Gabapentin (GBP), lacosamide (LCM), LTG, levetiracetam (LEV), oxcarbazepine (OXC), pregabalin (PGB), tiagabine (TGB), TPM and zonisamide (ZNS) are widely available for partial seizures. Rufinamide (RFN) has been licensed in Europe and the USA for adjunctive treatment of seizures in Lennox–Gastaut syndrome. Eslicarbazepine acetate (ESL) is licensed in Europe as adjunctive treatment for partial seizures with or without secondary generalization. Retigabine (RTG) has recently been approved for use in Europe and the USA (where it is called ezogabine) for the same indication. After 20 years of global experience, vigabatrin (VGB) has been approved in the USA for the treatment of infantile spasms and as add-on therapy for drug-resistant complex partial seizures. However, the use of VGB has also been markedly restricted because of reports of concentric visual field defects in up to 40% of patients. Stiripentol (STP) was licensed in 2001 for the adjunctive treatment of Dravet syndrome in Europe via the orphan drugs system. A similar arrangement has taken place in the USA for CLB in the treatment of Lennox–Gastaut syndrome. This drug has been available elsewhere in the world since the 1970s. The progress of felbamate (FBM) has been dramatically curtailed because of the unusual development of idiosyncratic life-threatening bone-marrow and liver toxicities. The advent of these newer agents has provided many more options in the management of refractory epilepsy, although whether overall outcomes have improved substantially is debatable.

Some of these AEDs – LEV, LTG, GBP, OXC and TPM – have also demonstrated efficacy as monotherapies in newly diagnosed epilepsy and have received approval for this indication in some countries. The pharmacological properties of these newer AEDs are highlighted in Table 5.4. Dosing information in adults and children is summarized in Tables 5.5 and 5.6, respectively.

Eslicarbazepine acetate (ESL) is a third-generation novel voltage-gated sodium-channel blocker. It is a pro-drug that is rapidly biotransformed to the (S)-entantiomer of licarbazepine. ESL is structurally similar to CBZ, but it is not metabolized to the active epoxide metabolite, which contributes to the latter's side-effect profile. Its precise mechanism of

75

TABLE 5.4

Pharmacological properties of modern antiepileptic drugs

Drug	Mode(s) of action	Indications (types of seizure/syndrome)
Eslicarbazepine acetate	Blocks fast-inactivated state of Na⁺ channel	Partial, GTCS
Felbamate	Various actions on multiple targets	Partial onset, Lennox–Gastaut
Gabapentin	Blocks high-voltage-activated Ca⁺⁺ channel	Partial onset
Lacosamide	Blocks slow-inactivated state of Na⁺ channel	Partial onset
Lamotrigine	Blocks fast-inactivated state of Na⁺ channel/other mechanisms	Partial, generalized, Lennox–Gastaut
Levetiracetam	Modulates synaptic vesicle protein 2A (SV2A)	Partial, GTCS, myoclonic
Oxcarbazepine	Blocks fast inactivated state of Na⁺ channel	Partial, GTCS
Pregabalin	Blocks high voltage-activated Ca⁺⁺ channel	Partial onset
Retigabine (ezogabine)	Opens Kv7 K⁺ channel	Partial onset
Rufinamide	Sodium-channel blockade/others	Lennox–Gastaut, partial onset
Tiagabine	Blocks synaptic GABA reuptake	Partial onset
Topiramate	Various actions on multiple targets	Partial, GTCS, myoclonic, Lennox–Gastaut
Vigabatrin	Inhibits GABA transaminase activity	Partial onset
Zonisamide	Various actions on multiple targets	Partial, GTCS, myoclonic

*As monotherapy. †Parameters for active metabolite 10-hydroxycarbamazepine. GABA, gamma-aminobutyric acid; GTCS, generalized tonic–clonic seizure; SV2A, synaptic vesicle 2A.

Absorption (bioavailability %)	Protein binding (% bound)	Elimination half-life* (hours)	Routes of elimination
Rapid (90)	40	13–20	Glucuronidation Renal excretion
Slow (95–100)	22–36	13–23	Hepatic metabolism Renal excretion
Slow (60)	0	6–9	Not metabolized Renal excretion
Rapid (95–100)	< 15	13	Hepatic metabolism 40% excreted unchanged
Rapid (95–100)	55	22–36	Glucuronidation
Rapid (95–100)	< 10	7–8	Non-hepatic hydrolysis Renal excretion
Rapid (95–100)	40[†]	8–10[†]	Hepatic conversion to active moiety
Rapid (90–100)	0	6	Renal excretion
Slow (60)	80	6–10	Hepatic metabolism Renal excretion
Slow (≥ 85)	34	6–10	Hepatic metabolism
Rapid (95–100)	96	5–9	Hepatic metabolism
Slow (80)	9–17	20–24	Hepatic metabolism Renal excretion
Slow (60–80)	0	5–7	Not metabolized Renal excretion
Rapid (95–100)	40–60	50–68	Hepatic metabolism Renal excretion

TABLE 5.5

Dosing guidelines for modern antiepileptic drugs in adults

Drug	Starting dose (mg/day)	Commonest dose (mg/day)	Maintenance range (mg/day)	Dosing interval
Eslicarbazepine acetate	400	800	800–1200	od
Felbamate	1200	2400	1800–4800	tds
Gabapentin	300–400	2400	1200–4800	tds
Lacosamide	100	400	200–600	bd
Lamotrigine	12.5–25*	200–400	100–800	od–bd
Levetiracetam	500	2000–3000	1000–4000	bd
Oxcarbazepine	150–600	900–1800	900–2700	bd–tds
Pregabalin	150	300	150–600	bd–tds
Retigabine[†]	150–300	900	600–1200	tds
Rufinamide	400	1600	400–3200	bd
Tiagabine	4–10	40	20–60	bd–qds
Topiramate	25–50	200–400	100–1000	bd
Vigabatrin	500–1000	3000	2000–4000	od–bd
Zonisamide	100	300	200–600	od–bd

*12.5 mg with sodium valproate (every other day in the USA); 25 mg as monotherapy. Also see Table 5.7 for schedules recommended for add-on or monotherapy use.
[†]Ezogabine in the USA.
od, once daily; bd, twice daily; tds, three times a day; qds, four times a day.

action is unknown, but it is thought to selectively target rapidly firing neurons by binding to site 2 of the inactive sodium channel.

Indications. ESL has been approved in Europe as adjunctive therapy for partial seizures with or without secondary generalization in patients 18 years of age or older. ESL tends to be better tolerated than CBZ with a lower potential for allergic rash and hyponatremia.

Dosage. The recommended starting dose is 400 mg once daily, increasing usually to 800 mg once daily after 1 or 2 weeks, thus

TABLE 5.6

Dosing guidelines for modern antiepileptic drugs in children

Drug	Starting dose (mg/kg/day)	Maintenance dose (mg/kg/day)	Dosing interval
Eslicarbazepine acetate*	–	–	–
Felbamate	15	30–45	tds–qds
Gabapentin*	20	20–40	tds
Lacosamide*	–	–	–
Lamotrigine			
– monotherapy	0.5	2–8	od–bd
– with valproate	0.15	1–5	od–bd
Levetiracetam	10	20–60	bd
Oxcarbazepine	5	10–50	bd–tds
Pregabalin*†	–	–	–
Retigabine*†	–	–	–
Rufinamide	see text		bd
Tiagabine*†	–	–	–
Topiramate	0.5–1 (od)	5–9	bd
Vigabatrin	40	50–150	od–bd
Zonisamide	2–4	4–8	bd

*Not approved for use in pediatric population.
†Not yet recommended for children under 12 years of age.
od, once daily; bd, twice daily; tds, three times a day; qds, four times a day.

offering fast titration. The dose can be titrated further to 1200 mg once daily. Limited safety information is available for patients over 65 years of age. No dose adjustment is needed in patients with mild-to-moderate renal or hepatic impairment.

Side effects. ESL is generally well tolerated. The commonest side effects are dizziness and somnolence. Other complaints during clinical trials have included headache, abnormal coordination, disturbed attention, tremor, diplopia, blurred vision, vertigo, nausea, vomiting, diarrhea and rash. Patients taking CBZ and ESL in placebo-controlled studies tended to report diplopia, abnormal coordination and dizziness more often than with other combinations. Hyponatremia occurs less frequently with ESL than with CBZ and much less frequently than with OXC.

Pharmacokinetics and drug–drug interactions. The effective steady-state half-life of ESL is 20–24 hours, which is longer than the single-dose half-life of 13–20 hours, allowing once-daily dosing. Peak plasma levels are reached after 1–4 hours and steady-state concentrations are attained in 4–5 days. Coadministration of ESL with PHT results in reduced ESL concentrations with increased PHT levels. Hence, the dosage of PHT may need adjustment if these drugs are used in combination. Like CBZ and OXC, ESL demonstrates an interaction with the combined oral contraceptive, accelerating the clearance of both hormonal components.

Felbamate (FBM) potentiates GABA activity and blocks voltage-dependent sodium channels as well as the ion channel at the N-methyl-D-aspartate excitatory amino-acid receptor.

Indications. FBM has demonstrated effectiveness both as monotherapy and add-on therapy for partial-onset seizures with or without secondary generalization in patients 14 years of age or older. It also has important efficacy as adjunctive therapy in the treatment of partial and generalized seizures (including atonic seizures) associated with the Lennox–Gastaut syndrome in children.

Dosage. Dosing should be initiated slowly and titrated over several weeks to minimize side effects. Doses of 1800–4800 mg daily in adults and 15–45 mg/kg daily in children are usually necessary for optimal seizure control. Routine monitoring of liver and bone-marrow function is recommended, but will not fully predict potentially fatal toxicity.

Side effects include insomnia, headache, nausea, anorexia, somnolence, vomiting, weight loss and dizziness. Clinical experience with FBM subsequent to its approval by the US Food and Drug Administration (FDA) showed a notable incidence of aplastic anemia and hepatotoxicity. As a result, the use of FBM is now largely restricted to patients with Lennox–Gastaut syndrome for whom the benefits of treatment outweigh the risks.

Pharmacokinetics and drug–drug interactions. In total, 25% of FBM is bound to plasma protein and approximately 50% is metabolized by the hepatic cytochrome P450 (CYP) system. Its half-life ranges from 15 to 24 hours. FBM increases serum concentrations of PHT, VPA and CBZ epoxide. Thus, dose adjustment of concomitant AEDs is usually necessary when FBM is introduced.

Gabapentin (GBP) was developed by adding a cyclohexyl group to GABA, which allowed it to cross the blood–brain barrier. Despite its structure, GBP does not bind to GABA receptors in the CNS. It appears to work by binding to the $\alpha_2\delta$ subunit of the neuronal voltage-gated calcium channels, inhibiting calcium flow and neurotransmitter release from presynaptic neurons.

Indications. GBP is approved as adjunctive therapy for partial seizures with or without secondary generalization in patients 12 years of age or older. It has also been licensed as monotherapy for these types of seizures in some countries. It may exacerbate myoclonic jerks and generalized absences. In addition, GBP is a useful drug for the treatment of neuropathic pain.

Dosage. Dosing should be initiated at 300 mg or 400 mg a day and increased in 300-mg or 400-mg increments every 1–3 days to the maximum tolerated dose using a thrice-daily regimen. The recommended dose range is 1200–2400 mg daily (900–1800 mg daily in the USA). However, many patients with drug-resistant epilepsy will need higher amounts (up to 4800 mg daily) for optimal seizure control.

Side effects are generally mild and transient. Drowsiness, ataxia, dizziness and nystagmus are the most common. Weight gain occurs in up to 5% of patients, particularly at higher doses. Flatulence, diarrhea and myoclonic jerks have also been reported. No idiosyncratic reactions or effects on bone marrow or hepatic function have been described.

Pharmacokinetics and drug–drug interactions. GBP is not metabolized in the liver, and it neither induces nor inhibits hepatic enzymes. Drug interactions, therefore, are not an issue with this agent. Its half-life is 6–9 hours. GBP is eliminated unchanged by the kidneys, so patients with renal insufficiency need lower doses and less frequent dosing. A useful serum concentration range has not been established.

Lacosamide (LCM) is a member of a group of functionalized amino acids synthesized to harness their anticonvulsant properties. Evidence suggests that the drug exerts its antiepileptic effect in a novel way – by enhancing the slow inactivation of voltage-gated sodium channels.

Indications. LCM is indicated as adjunctive therapy in the treatment of partial-onset seizures with or without secondary generalization in patients aged 16 years and older (17 years and older in the USA).

Dosage. The recommended starting dose is 50 mg twice daily, which should be increased to 100 mg twice daily after 1 week for maintenance. The maximum recommended dose is 200 mg twice daily (400 mg daily), although doses up to 600 mg daily have demonstrated efficacy in placebo-controlled clinical trials. LCM is also available as a syrup and intravenous injection. No dosage adjustment is needed in the elderly or in patients with mild-to-moderate renal or hepatic impairment. Outcomes with LCM may be better in patients treated with other AEDs that do not have a major pharmacological effect on sodium channels.

Side effects. Common problems include dizziness, headache, diplopia and nausea. Other reported adverse effects include vomiting, fatigue, blurred vision, poor coordination, somnolence, tremor and nystagmus. Minor prolongation in the PR interval has been observed in clinical studies and so LCM is contraindicated in patients with second- or third-degree atrioventricular block. The tablet form contains soy-derived lecithin in the coating, which may be a concern for some individuals with soy or peanut allergies.

Pharmacokinetics and drug–drug interactions. Oral LCM is completely absorbed with an elimination half-life of around 13 hours. Of the total dose, 40% is excreted unchanged in the urine. LCM does not inhibit or induce hepatic metabolic enzymes. There are no interactions, therefore, between LCM and the hormonal components of the oral contraceptive pill. Enzyme inducers such as PHT, PB, CBZ, rifampicin and St John's wort may reduce LCM concentrations.

Lamotrigine (LTG) selectively blocks the slow inactivated state of the sodium channel, thereby preventing the release of excitatory amino-acid neurotransmitters, particularly glutamate and aspartate. This mode of action does not explain its anti-absence and anti-myoclonic properties.

Indications. LTG appears to be effective across the complete range of seizure types, including partial seizures, the idiopathic generalized epilepsies and Lennox–Gastaut syndrome. It is licensed widely as add-on treatment for adults with drug-resistant epilepsy. Its use in children and as monotherapy in newly diagnosed epilepsy has been approved in a growing number of countries. Good results have been reported in patients with learning disabilities, who often have multiple seizure types. The ability of LTG to reduce interictal spiking may explain the improved alertness reported by some people taking the drug. Its efficacy may be enhanced when combined with VPA, although this combination is associated with higher rates of rash, tremor and teratogenesis. LTG may exacerbate myoclonic seizures in some patients, particularly those with severe myoclonic epilepsy. It is less effective than ESM and VPA for the treatment of children with typical absence only, without generalized tonic–clonic seizures (GTCS).

Dosage. LTG can be administered once daily as monotherapy or with VPA, or twice daily in patients taking enzyme-inducing AEDs. A low starting dose with a slow titration schedule will reduce the risk of rash, though this depends on concomitant medication (Table 5.7). Some patients respond to and tolerate doses exceeding 600 mg daily as monotherapy, or above 800 mg daily in combination with an enzyme-inducing AED. An equivalent high dose in VPA-treated patients would be 150–200 mg daily because of the extent of metabolic inhibition. A once-daily controlled-release formulation is now available in the USA.

Side effects include headache, nausea, insomnia, vomiting, dizziness, diplopia, ataxia and tremor. The drug seldom causes sedation. Rash complicates initial management in around 3% of

83

TABLE 5.7

Lamotrigine dosing and titration schedules

As add-on therapy	Concomitant antiepileptic drugs	
Adults		
	Valproate	Others
Weeks 1 and 2	12.5 mg daily*	50 mg daily
Weeks 3 and 4	25 mg daily†	50 mg twice daily
Maintenance	50–100 mg‡ twice daily	100–200 mg‡ twice daily
Children		
	Valproate	Others
Weeks 1 and 2	0.15 mg/kg	0.6 mg/kg
Weeks 3 and 4	0.3 mg/kg	1.2 mg/kg
Increments	0.3 mg/kg	1.2 mg/kg
Maintenance	1–5 mg/kg‡	5–15 mg/kg‡
As monotherapy	Adults	Children
Weeks 1 and 2	25 mg daily	0.5 mg/kg
Weeks 3 and 4	25 mg twice daily	1 mg/kg
Maintenance	50–100 mg‡ twice daily	2–8 mg/kg‡

*12.5 mg every other day is more common in the USA.
†12.5 mg daily is more common in the USA.
‡Higher doses can be tried if seizures persist and the patient's tolerance is good.

patients taking LTG as monotherapy, and in 8% of those already established on VPA. It is usually maculopapular and, in mild cases, may subside spontaneously without drug withdrawal. In a few patients, however, there is an accompanying systemic illness with malaise, fever, arthralgia, myalgia, lymphadenopathy and eosinophilia. Cases of bullous erythema multiforme, Stevens–Johnson syndrome and toxic epidermal necrolysis have also been reported. The risk of a severe skin reaction may be as high as 1 in 1000 adults and 1 in 100 children. Gradual introduction of LTG lessens the likelihood of rash,

84

so adherence to the prescribing guidelines should be strict. Preliminary results from large-scale pregnancy registries suggest only a small, dose-dependent risk of major fetal malformation associated with LTG monotherapy (4.5% with doses exceeding 300 mg daily). This risk may be considerably higher (up to 11%) when the drug is given with VPA.

Pharmacokinetics and drug–drug interactions. LTG does not influence the metabolism of lipid-soluble drugs, including other AEDs and warfarin. Co-prescription with the oral contraceptive pill results in reduction in the concentration of LTG and levonorgestrel. When used as monotherapy, the half-life of LTG approximates 24 hours. When it is given to patients already being treated with the enzyme-inducing agents CBZ, PHT or PB, the half-life falls to about 15 hours. VPA inhibits glucuronidation of LTG, prolonging its half-life to around 60 hours. Withdrawal of enzyme-inducing AEDs, therefore, causes a rise in the circulating concentrations of LTG, while discontinuing VPA produces a fall.

Serum concentrations of LTG fall dramatically during pregnancy, in patients starting an estrogen-containing oral contraceptive and in women just before the onset of menses. In these circumstances, concentration monitoring may be helpful in guiding LTG dose adjustment.

A pharmacodynamic interaction resulting in symptoms of neurotoxicity (headache, dizziness, nausea, diplopia, ataxia) is a common consequence when LTG is introduced in patients established on high-dose CBZ or OXC. This effect can be reduced by staggering doses of CBZ or OXC and LTG by 2–3 hours instead of administering them simultaneously. A pharmacodynamic interaction has also been proposed as the explanation for the marked tremor seen in some patients taking VPA and LTG in combination.

Levetiracetam (LEV) is an enantiomer of the ethyl analog of piracetam. It binds to synaptic vesicle protein 2A (SV2A), a protein involved in synaptic vesicle exocytosis, and releases a range of neurotransmitters.

Indications. LEV is approved for use in adults and in children aged 4 years and older. It has proven efficacy for drug-resistant partial seizures and a variety of generalized seizure types, including myoclonic jerks. It is licensed as initial monotherapy for patients with newly diagnosed epilepsy in Europe but not in the USA. A controlled-release formulation is available in the USA but not in Europe. An intravenous formulation has also been licensed in the USA for use in adults and in Europe for patients aged 4 years and older when oral administration is temporarily not feasible, such as immediately before, during and after surgery.

Dosage. In controlled studies, patients with partial seizures responded to 1000–3000 mg daily. Daily doses of up to 4000 mg appear to be well tolerated. Treatment can be initiated at 250–500 mg twice daily and titrated in 1000-mg increments every 2 weeks as tolerated and needed for seizure control. Seizures in some patients will be controlled on doses as low as 250 mg twice daily. Urinary excretion of unchanged drug accounts for approximately 60% of an administered dose, so patients with moderate-to-severe renal impairment will need lower amounts given at longer intervals.

Side effects. LEV is generally well tolerated. The most common side effect is sleepiness or somnolence. Some patients complain of headache, anorexia and nervousness. Behavioral problems such as agitation, aggression, emotional lability, hostility, psychosis, anxiety and depression are not uncommon, particularly in patients with a history of psychiatric illness. The patient and family should be warned about the possibility of aggression, particularly if the patient has a history of mental retardation or dementia. The risk of behavioral side effects may be reduced by adopting a slower titration schedule. Idiosyncratic skin rash with LEV has been rarely reported. Early data suggest that this drug may be safe in pregnancy.

Pharmacokinetics and drug–drug interactions. The major metabolic pathway for LEV is hydrolysis of the acetamide group to the inactive carboxylic derivative. Because its metabolism is independent of the hepatic CYP system, it has no clinically important pharmacokinetic interactions with other drugs, including oral contraceptives. Steady state is achieved after 2 days of twice-daily dosing. Children clear LEV faster than adults. In young adults, the half-life is 7–8 hours, compared with 10–11 hours in the healthy elderly, who have age-related diminished renal function.

Oxcarbazepine (OXC), the 10-keto analog of CBZ, is licensed worldwide. It is functionally a prodrug, being rapidly reduced in the liver to the active metabolite 10,11-dihydro-10-hydroxycarbamazepine. Principally, it prevents burst firing of neurons by blocking sodium channels, but it also modulates calcium and potassium currents.

Indications. OXC has a similar spectrum of efficacy to CBZ against partial and tonic–clonic seizures. It tends to be better tolerated than CBZ with fewer neurotoxic side effects.

Dosage. The recommended starting dose for OXC in adults is 150–600 mg daily in two doses. The dose can be titrated upwards as clinically indicated to 3000–4000 mg daily. A starting dose of 5 mg/kg daily in children over 3 years of age can be prescribed, increasing gradually to a maintenance dose of about 30 mg/kg daily. Patients already on CBZ may be switched immediately to OXC using a dosage ratio of 1.5 OXC to 1 CBZ. Particular care in immediate switching needs to be taken when the daily CBZ dose exceeds 1200 mg. Plasma concentrations of the clinically active metabolite of OXC increase linearly with dose. No studies, however, have attempted to relate elevated plasma levels to efficacy or toxicity.

Side effects most often involve the CNS and include drowsiness, dizziness, headache, diplopia, nausea, vomiting and ataxia. Rash occurs less frequently with OXC than with CBZ, but like CBZ, OXC has been implicated in rare cases of Stevens–Johnson syndrome and toxic epidermal necrolysis. OXC does not appear to produce blood dyscrasias or hepatotoxicity. Hyponatremia, which may be due to an antidiuretic hormone-like effect, is somewhat more common with OXC than with CBZ, although affected patients are rarely symptomatic unless the serum sodium level dips below 125 mmol/liter. There is no evidence that OXC is a human teratogen, although high doses produce malformations in rodents.

Pharmacokinetics and drug–drug interactions. OXC has no effect on its own metabolism, but it induces a single isoform of CYP, resulting in accelerated clearance of the hormonal components of the oral contraceptive pill.

Pregabalin (PGB) has an amino-acid configuration and is structurally related to GABA. Like GBP, it binds with high affinity to the $\alpha_2\delta$ subunit of neuronal voltage-gated calcium channels.

Indications. PGB is licensed as adjunctive treatment for partial seizures with or without secondary generalization. It is also approved for the treatment of neuropathic pain and, outside the USA, generalized anxiety disorder.

Dosage. The recommended starting amount is 50–150 mg daily in two to three divided doses. The maximum dose used in regulatory trials is 600 mg daily, which can be prescribed as 300 mg twice daily or 200 mg three times daily.

Side effects include dizziness, somnolence, asthenia, headache and ataxia. Many patients experience weight gain, particularly at high PGB doses. Peripheral edema has also been noted occasionally.

Pharmacokinetics and drug–drug interactions. The absorption of PGB is rapid, linear and almost complete. The short elimination half-life of 6–8 hours led to the use of twice- and thrice-daily dosing in clinical trials. PGB is excreted unchanged by the kidney and displays no pharmacokinetic interactions with any other drug, including all AEDs. Dosage adjustment is necessary in patients with substantial renal failure and in those maintained on hemodialysis.

Retigabine (RTG)/ezogabine (EZG) is a first-in-class potassium channel opener for the treatment of adults with partial epilepsy. The adopted name for the drug in the USA is ezogabine with retigabine being used across the rest of the world.

Indications. RTG/EZG is licensed as adjunctive treatment for partial-onset seizures with or without secondary generalization in adults aged 18 years and over.

Dosage. RTG/EZG is taken in three divided daily doses. The maximum starting dose is 300 mg (100 mg three times daily). Thereafter the total daily dose can be increased, as clinically indicated, by a maximum 150 mg every week according to individual patient response and tolerability. The effective maintenance dose is 600–1200 mg daily in most patients. No dose adjustment is required in patients with mild renal and hepatic impairment, but lower doses are recommended in patients with more severe organ dysfunction.

Side effects. A dose–response relationship seems to exist for dizziness, somnolence, tremor, gait disturbance, diplopia and constipation. Confusion, psychosis and hallucinations have also been reported in clinical trials. RTG/EZG has shown no consistent effect on bladder function, but hesitation, dysuria and, very occasionally, urinary retention have been reported in association with RTG/EZG administration. Caution is advised when RTG/EZG is prescribed in patients with a prolonged QT interval or in those taking other drugs known to prolong the QT interval; in such patients it is recommended that an electrocardiogram be recorded before treatment is initiated.

Pharmacokinetics and drug–drug interactions. RTG/EZG exhibits linear kinetics with a bioavailability of around 60%. Its elimination half-life approximates 8 hours, supporting thrice-daily administration. RTG/EZG does not induce or inhibit its own metabolism. PHT and CBZ will increase its clearance by around 30%. Population kinetics show no clinically relevant interaction with other AEDs. RTG/EZG does not alter the metabolism of the hormonal components of the oral contraceptive pill. Its administration may increase serum digoxin concentration.

Rufinamide (RFN) is a triazole derivative that reduces the recovery capacity of neuronal sodium channels after inactivation, thereby limiting action potential firing. Other unknown mechanisms of action are also likely given the drug's broad-spectrum antiepileptic properties.

Indications. RFN is licensed widely as adjunctive therapy for the treatment of seizures associated with Lennox–Gastaut syndrome in patients aged 4 years and older. Particular benefit has been demonstrated in reducing tonic–atonic seizures ('drop attacks'). The drug also may have efficacy in drug-resistant partial seizures with or without secondary generalization although it is not licensed for this indication.

Dosage. The initial daily dose in children weighing less than 30 kg and not receiving VPA is 200 mg in two divided doses. This can be increased by 200-mg daily increments to a maximum of 1000 mg

89

daily. Children weighing under 30 kg who are also receiving VPA should have the same starting dose, but with a reduced maximum maintenance amount of 400 mg daily. Older or heavier children and adults should be started on 200 mg twice daily, increasing as necessary to a maximum dose of 3200 mg daily. The formulation can be crushed and administered with half a glass of water.

Side effects. The most common adverse events reported during the clinical development program were headache, dizziness, fatigue and somnolence. Less common problems were nausea, vomiting, anxiety, insomnia and weight gain. Hypersensitivity reactions with fever, rash and lymphadenopathy are rare. Status epilepticus was reported during the clinical trial program.

Pharmacokinetics and drug–drug interactions. RFN is extensively absorbed with an elimination half-life of 6–10 hours. It undergoes hepatic metabolism primarily via hydrolysis, with little involvement of the CYP system. RFN concentrations are decreased by coadministration of CBZ, PHT, PB and PRM. Significant increases in RFN plasma levels can occur when the drug is given with VPA. RFN may reduce the clearance and hence increase the circulating concentrations of PHT. RFN has no clinically relevant effects on the levels of PB, CBZ, LTG, VPA or TPM. It does, however, induce the metabolism of ethinylestradiol and norethisterone, common components of the combined oral contraceptive pill.

Stiripentol (STP) enhances central GABAergic neurotransmission by increasing GABA release, thereby prolonging the inhibitory effect of GABA.

Indications. STP has been licensed via the European orphan drug system as an adjunctive treatment for severe myoclonic epilepsy in infancy (Dravet syndrome).

Dosage. The dose advised for children is 50 mg/kg/day given two or three times daily, preferably during meals, and increased as necessary to a maximum daily amount of 3500 mg. It is available as 250-mg and 500-mg capsules and sachets for an oral suspension.

Side effects. The most frequently reported adverse events in the clinical trials were drowsiness, slowing of mental function, ataxia, diplopia, anorexia, weight loss, nausea and abdominal pain. Asymptomatic neutropenia was occasionally observed.

Pharmacokinetics and drug–drug interactions. The bioavailability of STP is low and the drug undergoes saturation kinetics at therapeutic doses. Its effectiveness during adjunctive therapy probably depends on its inhibition of the hepatic metabolism of other AEDs, including PHT, CBZ, PB, VPA and CLB. A reduction of the dose of concomitant therapy, particularly CBZ and CLB, is often necessary, sometimes by as much as 50%.

Tiagabine (TGB) selectively inhibits the neuronal and glial reuptake of GABA, and thereby enhances GABA-mediated inhibition (Figure 5.4).

Indications. TGB is licensed globally for use as add-on therapy in drug-resistant partial epilepsy.

Dosage. TGB is available as 5-mg, 10-mg and 15-mg tablets, except in the USA, Canada and Mexico where 2-mg, 4-mg, 12-mg, 16-mg and 20-mg tablets of TGB are produced. Studies suggest a minimal effective dose of around 20–30 mg/day as add-on therapy in partial epilepsy. The dose range most extensively studied has been 32–56 mg/day, but some patients have demonstrated benefit with up to 80 mg daily. Treatment in adults is started with 4–5 mg once or twice daily, followed by weekly increments of 4–5 mg. A change to three-times-daily dosing is recommended when 30 mg or more is prescribed daily. TGB should be taken with food to avoid rapid rises in plasma concentration. Routine monitoring of plasma levels is not required.

Side effects include dizziness, asthenia, nervousness, tremor, impaired concentration, lethargy and depression. Weakness due to transient loss of tone can occur at high doses. The most common reasons for discontinuation of therapy are confusion, somnolence, ataxia and dizziness. In clinical trials, TGB-treated patients experienced similar rates of occurrence for rash and psychosis as those taking placebo. The safety of TGB in pregnancy is unknown, but it is not teratogenic in animals at therapeutic doses. Absence stupor and non-convulsive SE have been reported as rare side effects; these generally respond to treatment with benzodiazepines.

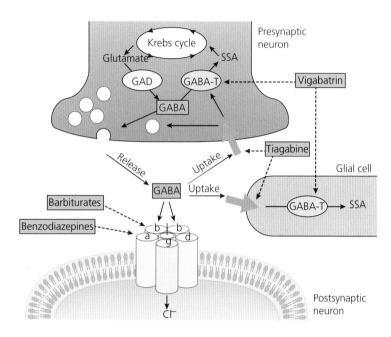

Figure 5.4 Effects of vigabatrin and tiagabine at the GABA$_A$ receptor. Vigabatrin inhibits GABA-T, which degrades GABA, and tiagabine blocks presynaptic neuronal and glial uptake of synaptically released GABA. GABA, gamma-aminobutyric acid; GABA-T, GABA transaminase; GAD, glutamic acid decarboxylase; SSA, succinic semi-aldehyde. Reprinted from Leach JP, Brodie MJ. Tiagabine. *Lancet* 1998;351:204. Copyright © 1998, with permission from Elsevier.

Pharmacokinetics and drug–drug interactions. TGB is rapidly and completely absorbed. Food reduces the rate, but not the extent, of absorption. It is extensively metabolized by hepatic oxidization via the CYP isoenzyme CYP3A. Because TGB does not induce or inhibit liver enzymes, concentrations of CBZ, PHT, theophylline, warfarin and digoxin are unaffected. VPA levels may drop slightly by an unknown mechanism. The half-life of TGB is 5–9 hours, falling to 2–4 hours when the drug is coadministered with hepatic-enzyme-inducing AEDs, such as CBZ and PHT. TGB shows linear pharmacokinetics that do not vary greatly in the elderly. Lower doses are required in patients with substantial hepatic, but not renal, impairment.

Topiramate (TPM) is a sulfamate-substituted monosaccharide that has multiple pharmacological actions involving blockade of sodium channels and high-voltage-activated calcium channels, attenuation of kainate-induced responses and enhancement of GABAergic neurotransmission. It also inhibits carbonic anhydrase, an effect that contributes to its side-effect profile.

Indications. TPM has proven efficacy against partial and tonic–clonic seizures. It also seems effective in myoclonic epilepsies, including some of the more severe syndromes of childhood. A useful effect on generalized absences has yet to be shown. However, it can provide benefit to patients with Lennox–Gastaut syndrome and possibly also infantile spasms. TPM has similar effectiveness to CBZ or VPA as monotherapy for partial and generalized seizures, and has received a monotherapy indication in some countries for newly diagnosed epilepsy. In addition to its indication for the treatment of epilepsy, TPM is also approved for migraine prophylaxis.

Dosage. Patients respond to TPM in doses ranging from 50 to 1000 mg daily. It is administered in two divided doses and should be introduced slowly. An initial dose of 25–50 mg daily can be increased by 25–50 mg every 1–2 weeks until a maximally effective and/or tolerated dose is achieved. The optimum dose for most patients with drug-resistant epilepsy appears to be 200–400 mg twice daily. Higher doses (400–800 mg daily) may be required in patients taking PHT or CBZ, with lower amounts (100–200 mg) often being successful in those taking non-enzyme-inducing AEDs. Some patients respond to doses as low as 50–100 mg daily, particularly if TPM is combined with LTG. Concentration monitoring of TPM is unnecessary. However, measurement of PHT levels may be necessary in patients who develop symptoms suggestive of toxicity. Women taking an oral contraceptive should use a formulation containing at least 50 μg of ethinylestradiol if the daily dose of TPM exceeds 200 mg.

Side effects related to the CNS include ataxia, poor concentration, confusion, dysphasia, dizziness, fatigue, paresthesia, somnolence, word-finding difficulties and cognitive slowing. The risk of neurocognitive side effects can be minimized by titrating the dose slowly. Anorexia and weight loss are common accompaniments of

TPM therapy. It increases the risk of nephrolithiasis tenfold and so should be avoided in patients with a history of kidney stones and in those taking calcium supplements or high-dose vitamin C. Sweating may be reduced in some children, leading to elevated body temperature. Acute glaucoma has been reported. TPM has been reported to be associated with an increased risk of facial clefts.

Pharmacokinetics and drug–drug interactions. TPM inhibits the metabolism of PHT in about 10% of patients. When used in doses over 200 mg/day, it can accelerate the breakdown of the estrogenic component of the oral contraceptive pill. PHT and CBZ induce TPM degradation, reducing its concentration by 40% or more.

Vigabatrin (VGB). The antiepileptic effect of VGB is mediated by suicidal inhibition of GABA transaminase, the enzyme responsible for the metabolic degradation of GABA (see Figure 5.4).

Indications. VGB is an effective add-on drug for patients with partial seizures with or without secondary generalization. It can worsen myoclonic jerks and generalized absences. Unfortunately, its usefulness has been severely limited by the development of visual field constriction in more than 40% of patients. This problem was first noted 8 years after the initial launch of the drug. As a result, VGB is only recommended as adjunctive therapy for partial seizures when there is no other alternative. However, VGB is still regarded by many pediatric neurologists as the treatment of choice for infantile spasms; more than 50% of children have been reported as spasm free after 1 week of treatment. Children with coexistent tuberous sclerosis often demonstrate a particularly favorable response. VGB is approved by the FDA for the treatment of infantile spasms and as add-on therapy in adults with drug-resistant partial-onset seizures.

Dosage. VGB is usually added to existing AED therapy, initially in a dose of 500 mg once or twice daily to allow tolerance to any sedation. If the patient complains of agitation or a thought disorder, the drug should be withdrawn immediately. Further increments of 500 mg or 1000 mg daily will depend on the clinical status of the patient. Seizures in most patients will respond to 2000–3000 mg daily. Few show further improvement at higher doses. Children should start treatment at 40 mg/kg daily, increased according to response up to 80–100 mg/kg daily. Infants with spasms may need as much as 150 mg/kg daily. When being discontinued, VGB should be tapered slowly, as abrupt cessation can produce a marked increase in seizures and can precipitate psychosis. Monitoring of VGB concentrations is unnecessary as the drug does not exhibit a useful concentration–effect–toxicity relationship.

Side effects. Tiredness, dizziness, headache and weight gain are the most frequent adverse effects with VGB. Some patients report a change in mood, commonly agitation, ill temper, disturbed behavior or depression. Paranoid and psychotic symptoms can develop. VGB can cause hyperkinesia and agitation in children. No idiosyncratic reactions have been reported. For patients in whom the benefit of VGB treatment is judged to outweigh the risk of visual field constriction (as discussed above), formal visual field monitoring should be performed every 6–12 months. There is no evidence that VGB is a human teratogen.

Pharmacokinetics and drug–drug interactions. VGB does not interfere with hepatic metabolic enzymes, but produces a small reduction in PHT levels of around 20% by an unknown mechanism.

Zonisamide (ZNS) is a sulfonamide derivative, chemically and structurally unrelated to other AEDs. It blocks voltage-dependent sodium and T-type calcium channels, and actively inhibits the release of excitatory neurotransmitters. Although probably not a major contributor to its pharmacological effect, a weak inhibition of carbonic anhydrase activity may contribute to its side-effect profile.

Indications. ZNS has proven efficacy for drug-resistant partial seizures. Evidence also suggests efficacy for infantile spasms and a variety of generalized seizure types, including tonic–clonic, tonic, atonic and atypical absence seizures. Pragmatic clinical studies suggest that ZNS may have important benefits in the treatment of myoclonic seizures, particularly in patients with juvenile myoclonic epilepsy (JME) and progressive myoclonic epilepsy. Apart from Japan and Korea, ZNS is licensed only as adjunctive therapy for partial seizures with or without secondary generalization. An application has recently been made for monotherapy use in Europe.

Dosage. The recommended initial dose for ZNS is 50–100 mg daily for adult patients, and 2 mg/kg/day for children in two divided doses. Because steady state is reached slowly, the dose should be increased at 2-week intervals to a target maintenance amount of 300–600 mg/day in adults and 4–8 mg/kg/day in children.

Side effects include anorexia, dizziness, ataxia, fatigue, somnolence, confusion and poor concentration. Gastrointestinal problems and loss of or decreased spontaneity have been described. Around 2% of treated patients develop renal stones that may resolve spontaneously. Allergic rash has also been reported particularly in patients sensitive to sulfonamides. In some children, sweating may be reduced leading to elevated body temperature. Neuropsychiatric symptoms, including depression, aggression, anxiety and mood swings, are occasionally associated with its use.

Pharmacokinetics and drug–drug interactions. The plasma half-life of ZNS is 50–68 hours, so a steady state is achieved in about 15 days. Children require higher daily doses than adults to achieve comparable serum concentrations because of faster clearance. Patients with renal dysfunction have lower rates of clearance. Enzyme-inducing AEDs, such as PHT, CBZ and PB, decrease the half-life of ZNS by approximately 50%. ZNS itself has no effect on the metabolism of other drugs. ZNS has a high affinity for erythrocytes, and this binding is saturable; the relationship between the dose and whole-blood ZNS concentration is therefore non-linear at high doses.

Antiepileptic drug treatment guidelines

Based on the findings from randomized controlled trials, various national and international guidelines have been developed for the use of AEDs as initial monotherapy for epilepsy. These guidelines focus on efficacy and effectiveness in the process of drug selection. Among the newer AEDs, the American Academy of Neurology and the American Epilepsy Society found evidence to recommend the use of GBP, LTG, OXC and TPM as monotherapies in newly diagnosed adolescents and adults with partial- or mixed-seizure disorders. In its 2006 guidelines, the International League Against Epilepsy (ILAE) included the older AEDs but adopted a stricter set of criteria in classifying evidence, particularly in the duration of measurement of efficacy, effectiveness parameters and statistical power. As such, it only recommends CBZ, PHT and VPA as initial monotherapies for partial-onset seizures in adults, and GBP and LTG for partial-onset seizures in the elderly. In a subsequently reported monotherapy study, LEV was non-inferior to extended-release CBZ, implying it should also fulfill the strict ILAE criteria for this indication. Other available guidelines include those from the UK (NICE) and Scotland (SIGN) (see page 140).

While these guidelines are extremely valuable in providing a working framework for the treatment of new-onset epilepsy, it is important to bear in mind that they focus on short-term evidence of efficacy and effectiveness alone. Other patient-related factors, discussed in Chapter 3, must also be considered when choosing the most appropriate treatment for the individual patient. Continuous advances in drug development also mean that these guidelines become rapidly outdated.

Key points – antiepileptic drugs

- Fifteen new antiepileptic drugs (AEDs) have been approved for the treatment of epilepsy since the late 1980s.
- AEDs differ substantially in their mechanisms of action, spectra of activity, and pharmacokinetic and side-effect profiles.
- This wider choice of AEDs permits pharmacological treatment to be better matched to the individual patient's circumstances.

Key references

Brodie MJ, Kwan P. New drugs for focal epilepsy in adults. *BMJ*; 2012; in press.

Brodie MJ, Perucca E, Ryvlin P et al. Comparison of levetiracetam and controlled-release carbamazepine in newly diagnosed epilepsy. *Neurology* 2007;68:402–8.

Chiron C. Stiripentol. *Neurotherapeutics* 2007;4:123–5.

Chiron C, Dulac O. The pharmacologic treatment of Dravet syndrome. *Epilepsia* 2011;S2(Suppl 2):72–5.

French JA, Kanner AM, Bautista J et al. Efficacy and tolerability of the new antiepileptic drugs I: treatment of new onset epilepsy: report of the TTA and QSS subcommittees of the American Academy of Neurology and the American Epilepsy Society. *Epilepsia* 2004;45:401–9.

French JA, Kanner AM, Bautista J et al. Efficacy and tolerability of the new antiepileptic drugs II: treatment of refractory epilepsy: report of the TTA and QSS subcommittees of the American Academy of Neurology and the American Epilepsy Society. *Epilepsia* 2004;45:410–23.

Glauser T, Ben Menachem E, Bourgeois B et al. ILAE treatment guidelines: evidence-based analysis of antiepileptic drug efficacy and effectiveness as initial monotherapy for epileptic seizures and syndromes. *Epilepsia* 2006;47:1094–120.

Glauser TA, Cnaan A, Shinnar S et al. Ethosuximide, valproic acid, and lamotrigine in childhood absence epilepsy. *N Engl J Med* 2010;362:790–9.

Glauser T, Kluger G, Sachdeo R et al. Rufinamide for generalized seizures associated with Lennox-Gastaut syndrome. *Neurology* 2008;70:1950–8.

Hitiris N, Brodie MJ. Modern antiepileptic drugs: guidelines and beyond. *Curr Opin Neurol* 2006;19:175–80.

Kwan P, Brodie MJ. Phenobarbital for the treatment of epilepsy in the 21st century: a critical review. *Epilepsia* 2004;45:1141–9.

Meador KJ, Baker GA, Browning N et al. Foetal antiepileptic drug exposure and verbal versus non-verbal abilities at three years of age. *Brain* 2011;134:396–404.

Mohanraj R, Brodie MJ. Measuring the efficacy of antiepileptic drugs. *Seizure* 2003;12:413–43.

National Institute for Health and Clinical Excellence. The epilepsies: diagnosis and management of the epilepsies in adults and children in primary and secondary care. *Clinical Guidance 137*. London: NICE, January 2012. http://guidance.nice.org.uk/CG137

Scottish Intercollegiate Guidelines Network (SIGN). *Diagnosis and management of epilepsy in adults. A national clinical guideline.* April 2003, updated October 20, 2005. www.sign.ac.uk/pdf/sign70.pdf

Stephen LJ, Brodie MJ. Pharmacotherapy of epilepsy. Newly approved and developmental agents. *CNS Drugs* 2011;25:89–107.

Epilepsy surgery

Surgery should be considered for patients with drug-resistant seizures because of the increased mortality and progressive cognitive and psychosocial morbidities associated with uncontrolled seizures over many years. There is emerging consensus that once drug resistance is demonstrated, patients should be promptly referred to a specialty epilepsy center that offers surgery. In some situations, such as catastrophic epilepsy in children, patients should be referred urgently because of the risk of severe developmental disability.

A case-by-case assessment is needed. In addition to results of diagnostic tests, the patient's and the family's perceptions of epilepsy severity despite optimal pharmacotherapy and their expectations for the future are key determinants in the decision to operate.

Types of procedure. The type of surgical procedure performed depends on the indication (Table 6.1). The most common procedure is anterior temporal lobectomy for hippocampal or mesial temporal sclerosis. In well-selected cases, 70–80% of patients can become seizure free, with a surgical mortality close to 0% and less than 5% significant morbidity (e.g. hemiparesis, hemianopia).

Some patients may be suitable candidates for a more limited resection known as amygdalohippocampectomy in which the epileptogenic hippocampus and amygdala are removed, while sparing the temporal neocortex.

Other potentially curative procedures include lesionectomy to resect discrete structural lesions such as glial tumors and vascular malformations. In a palliative procedure (e.g. hemispherectomy/ functional hemispherotomy, corpus callosotomy, multiple subpial transection), the focus of the seizure is not resected. Instead, the aim of the operation is to disrupt the pathways important for the spread of epileptiform discharges in order to reduce the frequency and severity of the seizures. Corpus callosotomy is a treatment option for patients

TABLE 6.1

Types of epilepsy surgery and their indications

Procedure	Indication
Anterior temporal lobectomy	Mesial temporal sclerosis
Focal resection	Partial-onset seizures arising from resectable cortex
Corpus callosotomy	Tonic, atonic or tonic–clonic seizures, with falling and injury; large non-resectable lesions; secondary bilateral synchrony
Hemispherectomy	Rasmussen's syndrome or other unilateral hemisphere pathology in association with functionally impaired contralateral hand
Subpial transections	Partial-onset seizures arising from unresectable cortex

with severe generalized epilepsy, particularly atonic seizures with frequent falls and subsequent injuries. Multiple subpial transection is performed when the epileptogenic lesion cannot be removed because of its close proximity to the eloquent cortex, while hemispherectomy is a more drastic procedure in which an extensively diseased and epileptogenic cerebral hemisphere is removed, or left in place but functionally disconnected from other brain structures.

Presurgical evaluation. There is no universally agreed protocol to identify potential surgical candidates. Presurgical evaluation aims to establish the presence of drug resistance, delineate the epileptogenic zone to be resected and demonstrate that its removal will not cause additional unacceptable neurological or cognitive deficits. In practice, the evaluation involves a number of processes.

- A thorough review of the patient's seizure history and AED trials.
- Sophisticated video-electroencephalogram (EEG) monitoring, which localizes the onset of a number of seizures that are typical for the particular patient.

- High-quality MRI with dedicated 'epilepsy surgery protocol' to increase diagnostic accuracy.
- Functional imaging such as single photon emission computed tomography or positron emission tomography, when necessary, to delineate a potential epileptogenic zone.
- Neuropsychological testing, including intracarotid injection of amobarbital or functional MRI, to define the laterality of language and memory functions.

Lobar excision may be carried out with a high probability of improvement when all of the following are satisfied:

- EEG monitoring shows that seizure onset is consistently and repeatedly from the same portion of one frontal or temporal lobe
- other investigations are consistent with this localization
- the identified area can be removed safely without permanent cognitive, sensory or motor deficit.

If scalp EEG data do not clearly identify the seizure focus, or if the neuroimaging and/or neuropsychological testing results are inconsistent with the ictal findings, 'invasive' electrodes may be inserted into the brain for further seizure recording, often guided by the results of functional neuroimaging (Figures 6.1–6.3). When monitoring shows that seizures arise from different sides of the brain on separate

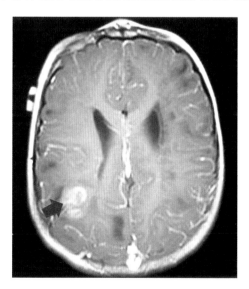

Figure 6.1 MRI scan of a patient with refractory epilepsy showing a heterogeneous lesion in the right parietal lobe (arrow).

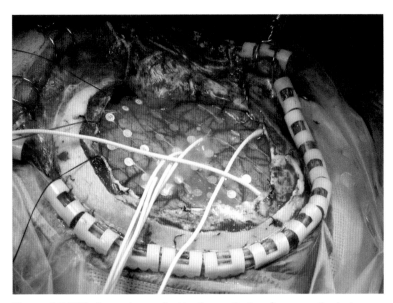

Figure 6.2 EEG electrodes applied to the cortical surface over the lesion intraoperatively to map out the area to be resected.

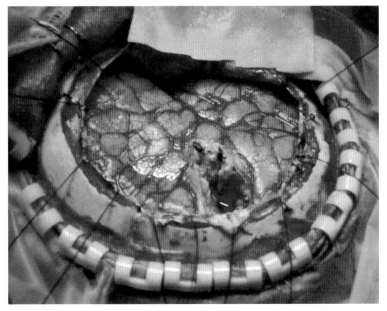

Figure 6.3 Patient in Figure 6.2 immediately after focal resection of the cortical lesion.

occasions, or are consistent with generalized seizures, lobectomy is unlikely to be of benefit. Intracranial electrodes also facilitate 'mapping' of eloquent cortex (areas with important functions such as motor and speech) so that it may be avoided during subsequent resection. Advances in neuroimaging techniques are reducing the need for invasive intracranial EEG recording.

Vagus nerve stimulation

The introduction of vagus nerve stimulation (VNS) in 1997 provided a non-pharmacological approach to epilepsy treatment. The VNS Therapy (Cyberonics, Texas, USA) system has been implanted in tens of thousands of patients worldwide. It comprises an implantable multiprogrammable pulse generator that delivers electrical current to the vagus nerve with the aim of reducing the frequency and/or severity of epileptic seizures. VNS is approved in the USA for use as adjunctive therapy for adults and adolescents over 12 years of age whose partial-onset seizures are refractory to AEDs. In Canada and the EU, VNS is indicated for use as an adjunctive therapy in reducing the frequency of seizures in patients whose epileptic disorder is dominated by partial seizures (with or without secondary generalization) or generalized seizures that are refractory to antiepileptic medications.

The VNS system (Figure 6.4) consists of:
• a programmable signal generator that is implanted in the patient's left upper chest
• a bipolar lead that connects the generator to the left vagus nerve in the neck
• a programming wand that uses radiofrequency signals to communicate non-invasively with the generator
• a hand-held magnet used by the patient or carer to turn the stimulator on or off.

The mechanism of action is unknown. It has no effect on hepatic metabolic processes, serum concentrations of AEDs or laboratory values. It does not have a deleterious effect on vagally mediated physiological processes (as assessed by Holter ECG monitoring), pulmonary function tests or serum gastrin levels.

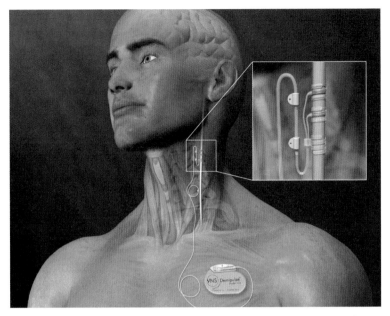

Figure 6.4 Vagus nerve stimulation (VNS) system in which the VNS pulse generator is linked by electrodes to the left vagus nerve in the neck. The enlarged section of the diagram shows how the ends of the flexible silicone leads are wrapped around the nerve. Reproduced courtesy of Cyberonics, Texas, USA.

Implantation and setup. The implantation procedure lasts approximately 1 hour with the patient under general anesthesia to minimize any possible seizure interference during surgery. Within the first 2 weeks after surgery, the output current is increased by the physician and adjusted to patient tolerance. A typical regimen consists of a 30-Hz signal frequency with a 500-microsecond pulse width for 30 seconds of 'on time' and 5 minutes of 'off time'.

Once programmed, the generator will deliver intermittent stimulation at the desired settings until any additional instructions are received or until the battery life is expended, typically after 6 years of operation with the latest model. In addition, the patient or a companion may activate the generator by placing the magnet over it for several seconds; in some patients, this may interrupt a seizure or reduce its severity if applied soon after the seizure onset.

Efficacy and tolerability. A number of severely affected patients treated with VNS have had clinically important seizure reductions of over 50%, and a few have become seizure free. Patients do not appear to become tolerant to the therapeutic effect induced by VNS.

Side effects are transient and include incisional pain, coughing, voice alteration, chest discomfort and nausea. Adverse effects related to stimulation are usually mild and almost always resolve with adjustment of the settings; they include hoarseness, throat pain, coughing, dyspnea and paresthesia. Patients may use the hand-held magnet to inhibit stimulation for side-effect management.

No cognitive, sedative, visual, affective, behavioral or coordination side effects have been reported; hence, the typical central nervous system problems associated with AEDs are conspicuously absent with VNS therapy.

Direct brain stimulation

Following the success of treatment for movement disorders, deep brain stimulation (DBS) is under active investigation as a non-pharmacological therapeutic modality for patients with medically intractable epilepsy who are not eligible for resective surgical procedures. Electrodes are inserted stereotactically to structures of interest and connected by extension leads to a subcutaneous battery-powered programmable stimulator to deliver intermittent signals of electric current. A variety of anatomic structures have been targeted. In the recently completed SANTE (Stimulation of the Anterior Nucleus of the Thalamus in Epilepsy) trial, bilateral stimulation of the anterior nucleus of the thalamus in patients with refractory focal epilepsy was associated with significant seizure reduction in the short term, resulting in approval of this device in Europe.

In another system, automated seizure detection is incorporated into an electric brain stimulator to form a closed-loop system so that stimulation is delivered to the epileptogenic zone when onset of ictal activity is detected. This system has undergone testing in a clinical trial and the results are under review by regulatory authorities.

Direct brain stimulation represents an exciting area of development but clearly further studies are needed to document its long-term

efficacy and safety in order to define its place in the clinical
management of epilepsy.

Ketogenic diet

The ketogenic diet is a restrictive high-fat, low-protein and very-low-
carbohydrate diet mostly given to children aged 5–10 years with
medically intractable epilepsy. There is much less experience to guide
its use in younger children, adolescents or adults. The diet mimics the
biochemical changes associated with starvation, which creates ketosis.
Its exact mechanism of seizure suppression remains unclear.

The diet was first developed in the 1920s but fell out of favor when
the choice of AEDs on the market increased. However, interest in the
diet has resurfaced since the early 1990s as it can be very effective in
patients in whom numerous drug trials have failed, and it does not
have the cumulative sedating effects of multiple AEDs.

Initiation and administration. The ratio of fat to carbohydrate and
protein ranges from 2:1 to 4:1 (Table 6.2). Meals must be carefully

TABLE 6.2

A typical day's meals for a child on a ketogenic diet*

Breakfast	Lunch	Dinner
60 g 36% heavy cream	60 g 36% heavy cream	60 g 36% heavy cream
20 g fruit	35 g vegetables	24 g vegetables
39 g eggs	19 g white tuna fish	31 g beef hotdog
22 g butter	24 g butter or margarine	14 g butter or margarine
		40 g sugar-free gelatin

*Information is based on a 5-year-old child of 18 kg bodyweight given a fat to
carbohydrate and protein ratio of 4:1.
Reprinted from Ballaban-Gil K. The ketogenic diet. In: Devinsky O, Westbrook
LE, eds. *Epilepsy and Developmental Disabilities*. Massachusetts: Butterworth-
Heinemann, 2002. Copyright © 2002, with permission from Elsevier.

chosen, with the quantities of foods strictly measured; this makes eating outside the home in schools or in restaurants difficult. Patients who require tube feeding can be provided with a liquid formula prepared from commercially available dietary powders. Patients are usually admitted for several days when the diet is initiated to monitor for any early complications such as hypoglycemia, and to educate the patient and family on how to administer the diet. Close collaboration between the patient and family, managing pediatrician and specially trained dietician is essential for successful implementation of the diet.

Efficacy and tolerability. The efficacy of the ketogenic diet has recently been demonstrated in a randomized controlled trial, confirming results of previous retrospective and prospective observational studies that showed that a greater-than-50% seizure reduction was seen at 1 year on the diet in approximately 50% of children with intractable epilepsy. In addition, a modified version of the diet (medium-chain triglyceride diet) appears to have similar efficacy. The diet seems to be effective in all seizure types. The major problem is adherence to the restrictive dietary regimen.

Dehydration, diarrhea and hypoglycemia may occur at the start of the diet. Common long-term side effects include weight loss or lack of weight gain, constipation and acidosis. Hyperlipidemia and renal stones are less common (6%). Rare cases of dilated cardiomyopathy, prolonged QT interval and hemorrhagic pancreatitis have been reported, but their causal relationship with the diet has not been established.

Other diets, including a low glycemic index diet and modified Atkins diet, are currently under study.

Alternative medicine
Herbal formulas have a centuries-old tradition in much of the world. Over-the-counter herbal and dietary supplements are increasingly popular with people in industrialized countries, especially patients with chronic illnesses such as epilepsy. In Japan, herbal medicines, called Kampo, are available by prescription from physicians.

Key points – non-pharmacological management

- Patients should be referred for presurgical evaluation after failure of two or more regimens using antiepileptic drugs (AEDs), particularly if they have a resectable lesion.
- Essential presurgical evaluation includes long-term video-electroencephalogram (EEG) monitoring, MRI with a dedicated protocol, and neuropsychological assessment for language and memory functions.
- Most patients (70–80%) with mesial temporal sclerosis can become seizure free after anterior temporal lobectomy.
- Vagus nerve stimulation is a therapeutic option for patients with drug-resistant partial-onset seizures, particularly those with non-resectable seizure foci.
- The ketogenic diet is effective adjunctive therapy for children with drug-resistant epilepsy.
- The ketogenic diet should only be used under expert medical and nutritional supervision.
- Up to one-third of patients with epilepsy take herbal or dietary supplements for general maintenance of health or the control of symptoms such as difficulty sleeping or depression. Thus, knowledge of the products taken by the patient may provide the clinician with information on AED side effects or comorbid mood disorders.
- Clinicians must take a thorough history from patients regarding the use of alternative medicines, and check reliable databases for information on safety as well as possible effects on seizure frequency and serum AED concentrations.

Surveys conducted in the USA and UK suggest that up to one-third of patients with epilepsy take herbal and/or dietary supplements, and that most of these patients do not discuss their herbal use with their physicians. Most patients take the alternative medicines for general maintenance of health or to control other symptoms – for example, valerian for difficulty sleeping, St John's wort for depression and

Ginkgo biloba for memory disturbance. Thus, the particular products taken by a patient may be a clue to that patient's side effects from AEDs or comorbid disorders.

Clinicians should take a thorough history regarding herbal and dietary supplements, and consult reliable databases for information on safety as well as possible effects on seizure frequency and serum AED concentrations. Certain herbs, such as St John's wort, can affect hepatic metabolism and therefore alter the serum concentrations of hepatically metabolized AEDs. In addition, anecdotal reports suggest that several herbal and dietary supplements, such as essential oils, evening primrose and borage, and stimulants such as ephedra (ma huang) and guarana exacerbate seizures.

Key references

Choi H, Sell RL, Lenert L et al. Epilepsy surgery for pharmaco-resistant temporal lobe epilepsy: a decision analysis. *JAMA* 2008;300: 2497–505.

Cross JH, Jayakar P, Nordli D et al. Proposed criteria for referral and evaluation of children for epilepsy surgery: recommendations of the Subcommission for Pediatric Epilepsy Surgery. *Epilepsia* 2006;47:952–9.

Ekstein D, Schachter SC. Natural products in epilepsy – the present situation and perspectives for the future. *Pharmaceuticals* 2010;3: 1426–45.

Engel J Jr, Wiebe S, French J et al. Practice parameter: temporal lobe and localized neocortical resections for epilepsy: report of the Quality Standards Subcommittee of the American Academy of Neurology, in association with the American Epilepsy Society and the American Association of Neurological Surgeons. *Neurology* 2003;60: 538–47; erratum 1396.

Fisher R, Salanova V, Witt T et al. Electrical stimulation of the anterior nucleus of thalamus for treatment of refractory epilepsy. *Epilepsia* 2010;51:899–908.

Lee PR, Kossoff EH. Dietary treatments for epilepsy: management guidelines for the general practitioner. *Epilepsy Behav* 2011;21:115–21.

Lyons MK. Deep brain stimulation: current and future clinical applications. *Mayo Clin Proc* 2011;86:662–72.

National Center for Complementary and Alternative Medicine. Using dietary supplements wisely. (USA). http://nccam.nih.gov/health/supplements/wiseuse.htm

Neal EG, Chaffe H, Schwartz RH et al. The ketogenic diet for the treatment of childhood epilepsy: a randomised controlled trial. *Lancet Neurol* 2008;7:500–6.

Neal EG, Chaffe H, Schwartz RH et al. A randomized trial of classical and medium-chain triglyceride ketogenic diets in the treatment of childhood epilepsy. *Epilepsia* 2009;50:1109–17.

Schachter SC. Vagus nerve stimulation therapy summary: five years after FDA approval. *Neurology* 2002;59(6 suppl 4): S15–20.

Spencer S, Huh L. Outcomes of epilepsy surgery in adults and children. *Lancet Neurol* 2008;7: 525–37.

Tyagi A, Delanty N. Herbal remedies, dietary supplements, and seizures. *Epilepsia* 2003;44:228–35.

Wiebe S, Blume WT, Girvin JP et al. A randomized, controlled trial of surgery for temporal-lobe epilepsy. *N Engl J Med* 2001;345:311–18.

Status epilepticus (SE) is a life-threatening medical emergency characterized by frequent and/or prolonged epileptic seizures. Community-based studies in the USA suggest the incidence may be as high as 50 per 100 000 people per year, peaking in children under 1 year of age and in adults over 60 years of age. With the aging of the population, it is likely that SE will become an increasingly important public health problem.

Traditionally, SE is diagnosed when the patient has continuous or repeated seizure activity without regaining consciousness for more than 30 minutes. This time frame is defined on the basis of decompensatory cerebral damage after 30 minutes of seizure activity when physiological changes fail to compensate for the increase in cerebral metabolism. In practice, however, most authorities would recommend emergency antiepileptic drug (AED) treatment when a seizure has lasted more than 5–10 minutes, excluding simple febrile seizures.

The most readily recognized type of SE is tonic–clonic SE, but it has been estimated that 25% of SE cases are 'non-convulsive' in nature. Diagnosis of the latter can only be established by concurrent EEG recording. Depending on the electrographic changes, non-convulsive SE is subdivided into complex partial and absence SE. SE is a neurological emergency that requires immediate treatment. SE may result from a variety of causes (Table 7.1), the commonest of which include non-compliance with antiepileptic medication, consumption of alcohol, metabolic problems, acute stroke and hypoxia.

Mortality/morbidity

Mortality and morbidity reflect the underlying cause and the physiological effects of prolonged convulsions, including hypertension, tachycardia, cardiac arrhythmias and hyperthermia. Mortality is as high as 10%, rising to 50% in elderly patients. Mortality is higher when SE is secondary to an acute insult (e.g. acute stroke, anoxia,

TABLE 7.1

Causes of tonic–clonic status epilepticus

With pre-existing epilepsy

- Poor compliance with medication
- Recent change in treatment
- Barbiturate or benzodiazepine withdrawal

Presenting de novo

- Presentation of a first seizure
- Alcohol or drug abuse
- Acute stroke
- Meningoencephalitis
- Acute head injury
- Cerebral neoplasm
- Demyelinating disorder
- Metabolic disorders (e.g. renal failure, hypoglycemia, hypercalcemia)
- Drug overdose (e.g. tricyclic antidepressants, phenothiazines, theophylline, isoniazid, cocaine)
- Inflammatory arteritides (e.g. systemic lupus erythematosus)
- Pseudostatus epilepticus

trauma, infections, metabolic disturbance). Conversely, SE resulting from a previous stroke, alcohol or AED withdrawal has a more favorable prognosis.

Management

A long duration of SE is associated with poor outcome. An effective management protocol should therefore be initiated immediately (Table 7.2). Any delay in treatment worsens the prognosis and reduces the likelihood of stopping seizures without having to resort to general anesthesia. The importance of a coordinated effort in the treatment of convulsive SE – involving ambulance technicians, emergency medicine

TABLE 7.2

Treatment protocol for uncomplicated convulsive status epilepticus

Time (min)	Action
0–5	• Diagnose SE by documenting recurrent convulsive seizures without recovery of consciousness in between, or continuous seizure for more than 5 minutes
	• Establish airway, and ensure adequate respiration, blood pressure and cardiac rhythm
	• Set up i.v. line with saline; draw blood for metabolic studies, AED levels and toxin screens
	• Administer thiamine and glucose if indicated
	• Give antibiotics when infection is a possibility
5–10	• Administer either lorazepam, 0.1 mg/kg at 2 mg/min i.v., or diazepam, 0.2 mg/kg at 5 mg/min i.v.
	• Repeat once if seizure continues after 5 minutes
	• Diazepam should be followed by i.v. fosphenytoin or phenytoin to prevent recurrence
10–30	• Administer phenytoin i.v. infusion, 15–20 mg/kg, no faster than 50 mg/min in adults and 1 mg/kg/min in children if SE persists
	• ECG and blood pressure monitoring during infusion
or	• Fosphenytoin i.v. infusion, 15–20 mg PE/kg, no faster than 100 mg PE/min
	• Pay special attention to respiratory depression

AED, antiepileptic drug; ECG, electrocardiogram; i.v., intravenous; PE, phenytoin equivalents; SE, status epilepticus.

specialists, medical intensivists and neurological specialists – cannot be overemphasized.

Most centers would initiate treatment with a benzodiazepine intravenously (most commonly lorazepam or diazepam), followed by phenytoin or fosphenytoin, or phenobarbital. If the seizure persists, the patient might be considered as having refractory SE and general

113

anesthesia would be warranted. Although not tested in randomized control trials, AEDs with intravenous formulations (e.g. sodium valproate, levetiracetam, lacosamide) are often used when first-line therapies fail. Table 7.3 lists the schedules for treating resistant SE, as discussed at the first London Colloquium on Status Epilepticus on behalf of the Taskforce on Status Epilepticus of the International League Against Epilepsy in 2007. In persistent SE, it is important to watch for potential complications including hypothermia, acidosis, hypotension, rhabdomyolysis, renal failure, infection and cerebral edema. An underlying cause should continue to be investigated. Treatment response should be monitored clinically and with EEG.

TABLE 7.3

Other pharmacological options for resistant status epilepticus in adults

Time (min)/stage	Treatment options: drug, dose (infusion rate)
10–30 min /stage 2 After benzodiazepine/ phenytoin or fosphenytoin administration (see Table 7.2)	• Sodium valproate, 20–30 mg/kg (10 mg/min); or • Levetiracetam, 30–70 mg/kg (500 mg/min); or • Lacosamide, 5–6 mg/kg (40–80 mg/min)
30–60 min/stage 3 After stage 2 treatment	Preferably in intensive care unit: • Phenobarbital, 20 mg/kg (100 mg/min); or • Midazolam, 0.2 mg/kg bolus (0.1–0.4 mg/kg/hour); or • Propofol, 3–5 mg/kg bolus (5–10 mg/kg/hour); or • Thiopental, 2–3 mg/kg bolus (3–5 mg/kg/hour)

Adapted from Shorvon SD et al. *Epilepsia* 2008;48:2177–84.

Seizure clusters

Some patients experience clusters of seizures (also called acute repetitive seizures) lasting from minutes to hours. Patients with frontal lobe epilepsy are particularly prone to clustering of seizures at night. Seizure clustering may occur around menstruation in women, or when patients do not take their usual AED therapy. In most cases, however, precipitating factors cannot be readily identified. These seizure clusters may not be defined as SE but nonetheless require therapeutic intervention. Acute treatment with a benzodiazepine such as clobazam after the first seizure can be given in an attempt to prevent further attacks. If the seizure cluster has occurred as a result of AED omission or dose reduction, reintroduction of the drug may be sufficient to abort it.

During a seizure cluster, oral therapy in a child may be problematic and intravenous access is usually unavailable or difficult. Rectal diazepam administered by parents or other caregivers may be effective in this situation. Rectal diazepam is absorbed more rapidly than rectal lorazepam or oral diazepam because of its high lipid solubility. A gel-containing prefilled unit-dose rectal delivery system is commercially available. The doses used in clinical studies (0.5 mg/kg for children aged 2–5 years, 0.3 mg/kg for children aged 6–11 years, 0.2 mg/kg for those over 12 years) were effective and well tolerated, and did not produce respiratory depression. The most common side effect was somnolence.

Buccal midazolam, recently made available in Europe, is being increasingly used instead of rectal diazepam. In adults and children over 10 years of age, 10 mg can be given and repeated once if necessary. Lower amounts can be used in younger children. Nasal formulations of benzodiazepines are under development.

Parents and caregivers must be adequately trained by knowledgeable healthcare professionals to be able to recognize seizure clusters, administer rectal diazepam or buccal midazolam, monitor the patient for potentially dangerous respiratory depression and summon emergency medical help when necessary.

Excessive use of rectal diazepam can result in rebound seizures.

Key points – status epilepticus and seizure clusters

- Status epilepticus (SE) can be convulsive or non-convulsive.
- Emergency treatment should be given when a convulsive seizure has lasted more than 5–10 minutes.
- Poor prognostic factors for SE include old age, acute symptomatic cause and long duration.
- Benzodiazepine administration, orally or rectally, can be useful in patients experiencing clusters of seizures.
- Buccal midazolam is being increasingly used in place of rectal diazepam for the treatment of seizure clusters (acute repetitive seizures).

Key references

Alldredge BK, Gelb AM, Isaacs SM et al. A comparison of lorazepam, diazepam, and placebo for the treatment of out-of-hospital status epilepticus. *N Engl J Med* 2001;345:631–7; erratum 1860.

Appleton R, MacLeod S, Maitland T. Drug management for acute tonic-clonic convulsions including convulsive status epilepticus in children. *Cochrane Data Syst Rev* 2008, CD00 1905.

Brodtkorb E, Aamo T, Henriksen O, Lossius R. Rectal diazepam: pitfalls of excessive use in refractory epilepsy. *Epilepsy Res* 1999;35: 123–33.

Chen JW, Wasterlain CG. Status epilepticus: pathophysiology and management in adults. *Lancet Neurol* 2006;5:246–56.

Haut SR, Shinnar S, Moshé SL. Seizure clustering – risks and outcomes. *Epilepsia* 2005;46: 146–49.

Koubessi M, Alshekhlee A. In-hospital mortality of generalized convulsive status epilepticus: a large US sample. *Neurology* 2007;69: 886–93.

McIntyre J, Robertson S, Norris E et al. Safety and efficacy of buccal midazolam versus rectal diazepam for emergency treatment of seizures in children: a randomised controlled trial. *Lancet* 2005;366:205–10.

Meierkord H, Boon P, Englesen B et al. EFNS guideline on the management of status epilepticus in adults. *Eur J Neurol* 2010;17: 348–55.

Meierkord H, Holtkamp M. Non-convulsive status epilepticus in adults: clinical forms and treatment. *Lancet Neurol* 2007;6:329–39.

Shorvon S. The treatment of status epilepticus. *Curr Opin Neurol* 2011;24:165–70.

Shorvon SD, Baulac TM, Cross H et al. The drug-treatment of status epilepticus in Europe: consensus document from a workshop at the first London Colloquium on Status Epilepticus. *Epilepsia* 2008;49:2177–84.

Treiman DM, Meyers PD, Walton NY et al. Veterans Affairs Status Epilepticus Cooperative Study Group. A comparison of four treatments for generalized status epilepticus. *N Engl J Med* 1998; 339:792–8.

Trinka E, Shorvon SD. The Innsbruck Colloquium on Status Epilepticus. Innsbruck, Austria, April 2–5, 2009. *Epilepsia* 2009;50(suppl 12):1–80.

Women of childbearing age

All doctors treating women with epilepsy should consider the following areas.

Contraception. Carbamazepine (CBZ), eslicarbazepine acetate (ESL), felbamate (FBM), oxcarbazepine (OXC), phenobarbital (PB), phenytoin (PHT), primidone (PRM), rufinamide (RFN), and topiramate (TPM) at doses over 200 mg daily all induce the metabolism of female sex hormones. This metabolism can alter the menstrual cycle and increase turnover of the components of oral contraceptive pills and depot formulations of steroid hormones (Table 8.1). The risk of breakthrough pregnancy is not insignificant.

TABLE 8.1

Interactions between antiepileptic drugs and oral contraceptives

AEDs that reduce serum levels of OC	AEDs with serum levels reduced by OC	AEDs that do not interact with OC
Carbamazepine	Lamotrigine	Benzodiazepines
Eslicarbazepine acetate	Oxcarbazepine	Gabapentin
Felbamate	Sodium valproate	Lacosamide
Lamotrigine		Levetiracetam
Oxcarbazepine		Pregabalin
Phenobarbital		Tiagabine
Phenytoin		Vigabatrin
Primidone		Zonisamide
Rufinamide		
Topiramate (> 200 mg daily)		

AED, antiepileptic drug; OC, oral contraceptive.

An oral contraceptive formulation containing 50 µg of estrogen, with subsequent adjustment depending on the presence or absence of breakthrough bleeding, can provide secure contraception, as can barrier methods. Other birth control measures must be taken until the pattern of menstruation has been stable for at least 3 months. Lamotrigine (LTG) reduces levonorgestrel levels by about 20%, which is a potentially significant decrease.

Levonorgestrel implants are contraindicated in women taking enzyme-inducing antiepileptic drugs (AEDs) as they have an unacceptably high failure rate. This is also likely to be the case with the progesterone-only pill. Medroxyprogesterone injections appear to be effective, though they need to be given more frequently than is usually recommended. The morning-after contraceptive pill can be used after unprotected intercourse. The effectiveness of the hormonal method of emergency contraception is reduced by enzyme-inducing drugs; a copper intrauterine device may be offered, or the dose of levonorgestrel should be increased.

Menstruation. Up to 20% of women with epilepsy have abnormal ovarian function, including anovulatory menstrual cycles and polycystic ovaries. These problems may be more common in patients treated with sodium valproate (VPA). Some women find that their seizures worsen mid-cycle or around menstruation, a phenomenon known as catamenial epilepsy. This exacerbation is thought to be a consequence of an imbalance between the proconvulsant estrogen and anticonvulsant progestogen concentrations. Manipulating the cycle with hormonal preparations is often unsuccessful, however, and may cause unwanted effects such as weight gain and depression. Another option is intermittent clobazam (CLB) for the few days just before and shortly after the onset of menstruation.

Pregnancy. The fertility of women with treated epilepsy is one-quarter to one-third lower than that of the general population. However, when women do conceive, most can expect to undergo uneventful pregnancies and deliver healthy babies. During pregnancy, metabolic processes change and close attention needs to be given to AED

119

concentrations. Total serum concentrations of some drugs will fall, particularly those of PHT (Figure 8.1) and LTG. Women whose epilepsy is well controlled usually remain seizure free during pregnancy and delivery. Conversely, those who continue to report seizures before conception may have increased seizures during pregnancy.

Before conception. Although it would be ideal to withdraw AED treatment in women contemplating pregnancy, for many this would result in recurrence or exacerbation of seizures that could be dangerous for both mother and fetus. If the criteria for discontinuation are met (see pages 56–7), the AED should be stopped over a suitable interval before conception. If AED therapy cannot be withdrawn completely, it should be tapered to a minimally effective dose of, if possible, a single drug. In addition, supplemental folic acid, 4–5 mg daily, should be started before conception in an attempt to prevent neural tube defects. Folate treatment should be continued for the first 5 weeks of gestation, and current advice is to continue taking it at least until the end of week 12. These and other guidelines for managing epilepsy in women who are contemplating pregnancy are set out in Table 8.2.

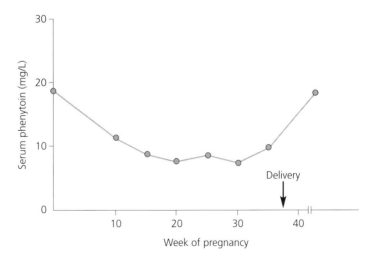

Figure 8.1 Serum phenytoin concentrations during pregnancy and delivery in a woman taking an established dose of 300 mg daily.

TABLE 8.2

Guidelines for managing epilepsy in women contemplating pregnancy

- After thorough discussion of the pros and cons with the woman, attempt AED withdrawal before conception if criteria are met
- If AED withdrawal is unsuitable (or the woman is unwilling to attempt it), review the regimen before conception, aiming for monotherapy (if possible) with the lowest effective dose of AED; stress the importance of planned pregnancy
- Discuss the risks of seizure exacerbation as well as fetal loss, teratogenesis and development delay with the patient and her partner
- Ensure potential mothers appreciate that by the time pregnancy is confirmed, possible teratogenesis is well under way and any damage may already have been done
- Discuss available antenatal screening and the need for frequent AED measurements during pregnancy and for at least 8 weeks after delivery
- Prescribe folic acid, 4–5 mg daily, before conception and continue at least until the 12th week of gestation
- Point out the potential risk of hemorrhagic disorder in the newborn and consider the need for oral vitamin K during the last few weeks of pregnancy in women taking enzyme-inducing AEDs
- Discuss the chance of the baby developing epilepsy; children born to mothers with epilepsy have a threefold increased risk of later seizures. While there may be risk of paternal transfer for some of the genetically transmitted epilepsy syndromes, there is no such risk for the common epilepsies
- Advise the patient about the need for strict AED compliance and adequate sleep throughout pregnancy
- Document each of the above in the patient's medical record

AED, antiepileptic drug.

Fetal health. The incidence of minor and major fetal malformations increases in women with epilepsy, even if they are untreated. Commonly quoted figures are 3–6% for women with epilepsy compared with 2–3% in the general population. The risk increases disproportionately with the number of AEDs taken, being approximately 3% for one drug (similar to background risk), 5% for two, 10% for three and over 20% in women taking more than three AEDs (Figure 8.2). A syndrome initially ascribed to hydantoins including PHT (fetal hydantoin syndrome), but now known to occur with other AEDs including CBZ and VPA, consists of facial dimorphism, cleft lip and palate, cardiac defects, digital hypoplasia and nail dysplasia.

There are no clear data indicating differences in safety among PHT, CBZ, PB and PRM. Current evidence suggests that the risk of major congenital malformations is two to four times higher with the use of VPA than with other AEDs such as CBZ and LTG. Absolute rates have ranged from 6% to 11%, although the risk may be minimized by keeping daily doses at or below 1000 mg. High-dose exposure to VPA in utero may impair later cognitive function. The teratogenic risk associated with LTG monotherapy is low and is similar to that associated with CBZ, although preliminary data suggest the possibility of greater risk of major malformations at higher dosage. There are still insufficient data regarding the safety of other modern AEDs.

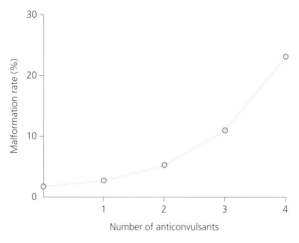

Figure 8.2 Relationship between number of antiepileptic drugs taken during the first trimester of pregnancy and the likelihood of fetal malformation. Data from Nakane Y et al. *Epilepsia* 1980;21:663–80.

After birth. The older enzyme-inducing AEDs (CBZ, PHT, PB and PRM) can cause transient and reversible deficiency in vitamin K1-dependent clotting factors in the neonate. The risk of intracerebral hemorrhage increases if the birth is traumatic. Accordingly, some clinicians believe that babies at risk should receive intramuscular vitamin K1 immediately after birth, and mothers should take oral vitamin K1, 10 mg daily, for the last few weeks of pregnancy.

After delivery, all mothers should be encouraged to breastfeed their babies. The concentrations of PHT, CBZ and VPA in breast milk are low and not usually harmful. PB, PRM and LTG can accumulate in the breastfed baby because of slow elimination. Gabapentin (GBP) and vigabatrin (VGB) are unlikely to accumulate in infants as these AEDs are excreted mainly unchanged in the urine. There are few data relating to the other newer AEDs. As a general rule, if the baby is noted to be drowsy or sedated, breastfeeding should be alternated with bottle feeding or stopped altogether.

Pregnancy registries. The Antiepileptic Drug Pregnancy Registry was established in the USA in 1996 to determine prospectively the risk of major malformations from AEDs. Women with epilepsy who become pregnant should call the toll-free number (1 888 233 2334) to enroll. Physicians cannot enroll patients; the woman herself must call as part of the informed consent process. There are three brief interviews: an initial 15 minutes, 5 minutes at 7 months' gestation and 5 minutes 2–4 weeks after birth.

In Europe, a similar project is under way. This registry requires input from the attending clinician and not the patient. The European Registry of Antiepileptic Drugs and Pregnancy (EURAP) is a consortium of independent research groups that have agreed on a common protocol for a prospective assessment of pregnancy outcome. The registry has now expanded beyond Europe to include Australia, Japan and other Asian countries. All physicians who care for women taking AEDs during pregnancy are invited to contribute. They can contact their individual national coordinators or the central project commission via dbattino@istituto-besta.it. There is also an active prospective pregnancy register in the UK.

Elderly patients

Old age is now the most common time in life to develop epilepsy. Approximately 1.5% of the population over the age of 70 years is diagnosed with active epilepsy. The number of elderly people diagnosed with epilepsy is set to rise further with the aging of the population. Nearly all de-novo seizures in elderly people are partial-onset with or without secondary generalization. Underlying factors can be identified in a greater proportion of elderly patients than younger patients, and include cerebrovascular disease, dementia and tumor. New-onset idiopathic syndromes are rare.

Diagnosis of epilepsy can be challenging and may depend on a witnessed event. Complex partial seizures presenting as confusion may be misdiagnosed as psychiatric symptoms. Postictal confusion can be prolonged in the elderly and may contribute to physical injury sustained during a seizure.

AEDs are the mainstay of treatment, and are effective in most patients. Complete seizure control can be expected in more than 70% of elderly patients. A subgroup, often with progressive neurodegenerative disease, will continue to have seizures despite all attempts at pharmacological prevention. Elderly patients are particularly sensitive to the adverse effects of AEDs, possibly because of age-related pharmacokinetic changes caused by the delay in gastric emptying, reduction in body fat, and decreased hepatic metabolism and renal elimination. Low doses are generally recommended in the elderly in order to minimize adverse effects.

The patient, and often the spouse and children, must be convinced of the need for lifelong treatment. Sympathetic explanation and assured support will help an elderly person regain their self-confidence after epilepsy has been diagnosed and AED treatment established. Choice of drug depends on the side-effect and interaction profiles. Drugs with a high propensity for neurotoxicity should be avoided (see Table 4.5, page 48).

In patients with multiple concomitant medications, AEDs that do not produce pharmacokinetic interactions are the preferred choice (see Table 4.6, page 50). Few clinical trials of AEDs have been performed specifically in the elderly. Double-blind trials support the newer agents LTG and GBP over CBZ for the treatment of partial seizures and generalized tonic–clonic seizures (GTCS), primarily because they produce fewer neurotoxic side effects. Levetiracetam (LEV) is a suitable alternative as it is also well tolerated in this population and is implicated in fewer drug interactions than is CBZ or PHT.

Teenagers

Some types of epilepsy, such as the idiopathic syndromes juvenile myoclonic epilepsy (JME) and GTCS on awakening, are most likely to manifest during the teenage years. Sleep deprivation, photosensitivity and major stresses such as school examinations are common triggers. Partial seizures can also present during the teenage years, either de novo or as a recurrence of a dormant childhood condition such as mesial temporal sclerosis.

Children who develop epilepsy should be re-evaluated during their teenage years, and AED levels should be monitored. At puberty, hepatic metabolism slows to a rate similar to that in adults, which may lead to a rise in circulating AED concentrations. AED doses may, therefore, need to be reduced as a child grows older. However, such a rise is often offset by a teenage growth spurt. Falling AED levels may indicate imperfect compliance, a common occurrence in this age group.

The teenage years are an appropriate time for counseling on contraception, clarifying the possible side effects of AEDs, and predicting prognosis and eventual drug withdrawal.

Driving, social interactions and career advice are other issues that doctors caring for teenagers with epilepsy must address (see Chapter 9).

Patients with learning disabilities

Epilepsy has the highest prevalence in people with learning disabilities, ranging from 5% in mildly affected individuals to 75% in those with coexisting severe cerebral palsy or postnatal brain injury. Diagnosis relies heavily on an accurate description of events, as routine investigations are rarely helpful. Tonic–clonic seizures are common, but many patients also have partial and other generalized seizure types. The clinical picture is often complicated by stereotypies and behavioral disorders. Co-prescription of antipsychotic drugs may further reduce the seizure threshold.

Before the doctor's first visit, a great deal of useful information can be obtained from a home assessment by a specialist epilepsy nurse following an agreed protocol.

The home assessment should include:
- description of the episodes
- evaluation of IQ
- details of concomitant medication
- previous and current AED treatment
- circulating AED levels if appropriate
- details of the carer's concerns and so on.

Home video recordings can help to confirm or refute the diagnosis of epilepsy. At the outset, a management plan, including outcome aims, should be formulated with the full involvement of the carer(s) and family. Numbers and doses of AEDs should be minimized as much as possible. Attention should be paid not only to seizure frequency and severity, but also to behavior, mood, appetite, communication, cooperation, alertness and sleep pattern. Broad-spectrum AEDs, such as VPA, LTG, TPM, zonisamide and LEV, should be the preferred choice, and barbiturates and benzodiazepines should be avoided. The endpoint need not always be freedom from seizures, but perhaps better control accompanied by improved alertness, mood and cooperation.

Key points – specific populations

- Oral contraceptives containing at least 50 μg of estrogen should be used when coadministered with carbamazepine, eslicarbazepine acetate, felbamate, oxcarbazepine, phenobarbital, phenytoin, primidone and rufinamide, and topiramate at doses over 200 mg daily, because these drugs induce the metabolism of female sex hormones.
- Intermittent clobazam just before and shortly after the onset of menstruation can be used in women who experience catamenial seizures.
- The risk of major malformations in babies exposed in utero seems to be greater with sodium valproate (VPA) than with other AEDs.
- AED treatment is continued when necessary during pregnancy because seizures, especially convulsive seizures, are more harmful to the mother and fetus than the drugs themselves; however, treatment should be tapered to a minimally effective dose before pregnancy, if possible to a single AED.
- Supplemental folic acid, 4–5 mg daily, should be administered before conception and continued at least until the end of week 12 of gestation.
- A witness's account is particularly important for the correct diagnosis of epilepsy in the elderly, in whom the presentation of seizures is often subtle.
- Low doses of AEDs are recommended in the elderly in order to minimize adverse effects, particularly neurotoxicity. Preferred choices include lamotrigine (LTG) and levetiracetam (LEV).
- The teenage years are an appropriate time for counseling on contraception and other lifestyle issues including driving, social interactions and careers.
- Broad-spectrum AEDs (e.g. VPA, LTG, TPM, LEV, zonisamide) should be the treatment of choice in people with learning difficulties; barbiturates and benzodiazepines should be avoided.

Key references

Brodie MJ, Elder AT, Kwan P. Epilepsy in later life. *Lancet Neurol* 2009;8:1019–30.

Brodie MJ, Kwan P. Epilepsy in the elderly. *BMJ* 2005;331:1317–22.

Brodie MJ, Overstall PW, Giorgi L; UK Lamotrigine Elderly Study Group. Multicentre, double-blind, randomised comparison between lamotrigine and carbamazepine in elderly patients with newly diagnosed epilepsy. *Epilepsy Res* 1999;37:81–7.

Foldvary-Schaefer N, Falcone T. Catamenial epilepsy: pathophysiology, diagnosis, and management. *Neurology* 2003; 61(6 suppl 2):S2–15.

Hannah JA, Brodie MJ. Epilepsy and learning disabilities – a challenge for the next millennium. *Seizure* 1998;7:3–13.

Harden CL, Hopp J, Ting TY et al. Practice parameter update: management issues for women with epilepsy – focus on pregnancy (an evidence-based review). Obstetric complications and change in seizure frequency. *Epilepsia* 2009;50: 1247–55.

Harden CL, Meador KJ, Pennell PB et al. Practice parameter update: management issues for women with epilepsy – focus on pregnancy (an evidence-based review). Teratogenesis and perinatal outcomes. *Epilepsia* 2009;50: 1229–36.

Harden CL, Pennell PB, Koppel BS et al. Practice parameter update: management issues for women with epilepsy – focus on pregnancy (an evidence-based review). Vitamin K, folic acid, blood levels and breastfeeding. *Epilepsia* 2009;50: 1237–46.

Jentink J, Dolk H, Loane MA et al. Intrauterine exposure to carbamazepine and specific congenital malformations: systematic review and case-control study. *BMJ* 2010;341:c6581.

Meador KJ, Baker GA, Browning N et al. Cognitive function at 3 years of age after fetal exposure to antiepileptic drugs. *N Engl J Med* 2009;360:1597–605.

Meador KJ, Pennell PB, Harden CL et al. Pregnancy registries in epilepsy: a consensus on health outcomes. *Neurology* 2008;71:1109–17.

Morrow J, Russell A, Guthrie E et al. Malformation risks of antiepileptic drugs in pregnancy: a prospective study from the UK Epilepsy and Pregnancy register. *J Neurol Neurosurg Psychiatry* 2006;77:193–8.

O'Brien MD, Guillebaud J. Contraception for women with epilepsy. *Epilepsia* 2006;47: 1419–22.

Palac S, Meador KJ. Antiepileptic drugs and neurodevelopment: an update. *Curr Neurol Neurosci Rep* 2011;11:423–7.

Perucca E. Clinically relevant drug interactions with antiepileptic drugs. *Br J Clin Pharmacol* 2006;61: 246–55.

Rowan AJ, Ramsay RE, Collins JF et al. New onset geriatric epilepsy: a randomized study of gabapentin, lamotrigine, and carbamazepine. *Neurology* 2005;64:1868–73.

Saetre E, Perucca E, Isojarvi J et al. An international multicentre randomized double-blind controlled trial of lamotrigine and sustained-release carbamazepine in the treatment of newly diagnosed epilepsy. *Epilepsia* 2007;48: 1292–302.

Tomson T, Perucca E, Battino D. Navigating toward fetal and maternal health: the challenge of treating epilepsy in pregnancy. *Epilepsia* 2004;45:1171–5.

Tomson T, Battino D, Bonizzoni E et al. Dose-dependent risk of malformations with antiepileptic drugs. An analysis of data from the EURAP epilepsy and pregnancy registry. *Lancet Neurol* 2011;10: 609–17.

Psychiatric comorbidities

Nearly 1 in 3 patients reports significant concern about their mood. Not surprisingly then, mood states and psychiatric comorbidities substantially contribute to the quality of life of patients with epilepsy. The three most common psychiatric comorbidities in patients with epilepsy are depression, anxiety and psychosis.

Depression is the most prevalent psychiatric condition in patients with epilepsy – up to 55% of patients in some studies – and has a greater negative impact on quality of life than seizure-specific variables such as seizure frequency and severity.

Depression is under-recognized and, when diagnosed, often undertreated. Depression associated with epilepsy differs clinically from depressive disorders in non-epileptic patients. Accordingly, symptoms of depression in patients with epilepsy often fail to meet the diagnostic criteria for affective disorders set out in the American Psychiatric Association's Diagnostic and Statistical Manual of Mental Disorders, fourth edition (DSM IV). Diagnosis may be further complicated if the patient minimizes their psychiatric symptoms, or if the clinician does not inquire about psychiatric symptoms or considers depression to be part of the normal adaptation to the diagnosis of epilepsy. Clinicians often inadequately treat depression because they are concerned that antidepressant therapy will increase seizure frequency. The consequence of underdiagnosis and undertreatment can be fatal. The overall suicide rate in depressed patients with epilepsy is five times higher than that in the general population and as much as 25 times higher in patients with complex partial seizures of temporal lobe origin.

Patients experience depression most often interictally as a chronic, waxing and waning disorder, usually in association with variable levels of irritability and emotionality. Some patients experience depression during a simple partial seizure (ictal depression) or during the postictal state.

Before therapy is initiated, iatrogenic causes should be excluded. Antiepileptic drug (AED) treatment can be contributory, especially phenobarbital (PB), primidone (PRM), vigabatrin (VGB), topiramate (TPM), levetiracetam (LEV) and zonisamide (ZNS). Conversely, depression that follows the discontinuation of an AED with mood-stabilizing properties (e.g. lamotrigine [LTG]) can also be treated by reinstituting the AED.

Few controlled trials of antidepressants have been conducted in patients with epilepsy and depression. Selective serotonin-reuptake inhibitors (SSRIs) are first-line treatments, especially citalopram and sertraline, which have minimal pharmacokinetic interactions with AEDs. Tricyclic antidepressants (TCAs) can be given as second-line therapy. Monoamine oxidase inhibitors and non-TCAs are probably best avoided. Clomipramine and lithium are more likely to worsen seizure frequency than other antidepressants. Electroconvulsive therapy is not absolutely contraindicated in patients with epilepsy but should be reserved for medication-resistant depression. In addition to antidepressants, contributing psychosocial factors should be sought and addressed by qualified professionals (see *Fast Facts: Depression*).

Anxiety is the second most common psychiatric condition in patients with epilepsy, with a prevalence of up to 50% in some studies. Anxiety markedly compromises quality of life and psychosocial functioning, even more so than depression in one study. Ictal anxiety may be mistaken for a panic disorder. Patients experience anxiety most commonly interictally in the form of a generalized anxiety disorder. Severity of anxiety does not necessarily correlate with seizure frequency. SSRIs and benzodiazepines are most often used, though no controlled studies in patients with epilepsy have been reported. Some AEDs, such as sodium valproate (VPA), gabapentin (GBP) and pregabalin (PGB), have anti-anxiety properties (see *Fast Facts: Anxiety, Panic and Phobias*).

Psychosis. The incidence of psychosis varies according to the epilepsy syndrome, from 3.3% in patients with idiopathic generalized epilepsy to 14% in patients with temporal lobe epilepsy. Additionally, it correlates with epilepsy severity: psychosis occurs in 0.6–7% of patients with epilepsy in the community and 19–27% of patients with epilepsy who require hospitalization.

Ictal psychosis presents as hallucinations or delusions. Symptoms are usually self-limiting and can be mistaken for schizophrenia or mania, but unlike a primary psychiatric disorder are associated with a pattern of non-convulsive status epilepticus on electroencephalogram (EEG) recording. Postictal psychosis generally begins years after the onset of epilepsy. The typical pattern is a cluster of complex partial seizures, followed by a lucid postictal period. In turn, this lucid period is followed by affective symptoms together with grandiose and religious delusions, as well as simple auditory hallucinations. Patients with bilateral seizure foci, bilateral limbic lesions and clusters of complex partial seizures are at particularly high risk.

Interictal psychosis manifests as delusions and hallucinations; disorganized behavior and thought disorders may also occur. Compared with patients with schizophrenia, patients with interictal psychosis have an absence of negative symptoms, better premorbid state, less deterioration of personality and better response to pharmacotherapy.

There are no controlled trials of antipsychotic or atypical antipsychotic medications in patients with epilepsy and psychosis. Haloperidol, molindone, fluphenazine, perphenazine and risperidone appear less likely to worsen seizure frequency than clozapine and loxapine. Some AEDs, such as TPM, VGB and LEV, can occasionally produce psychotic reactions in susceptible patients.

Drug interactions

Selective serotonin-reuptake inhibitors, especially fluoxetine and paroxetine, may increase serum concentrations of carbamazepine (CBZ) and phenytoin (PHT). These drugs also elevate serum concentrations of TCAs.

Tricyclic antidepressants. Serum concentrations of TCAs (which are metabolized by the 2D6 hepatic isoenzyme) are generally reduced by hepatic enzyme-inducing AEDs such as CBZ, PHT, PB and PRM.

Conversely, VPA inhibits the metabolism of TCAs and may increase their circulating concentrations.

Antipsychotics. Most antipsychotic drugs, including haloperidol, perphenazine, chlorpromazine, thioridazine, thiothixene and risperidone, are metabolized by the cytochrome P450 2D6 and/or 3A4 hepatic isoenzymes and therefore their serum concentrations are lowered by hepatic enzyme-inducing AEDs such as CBZ, PHT, PB and PRM, and increased by VPA.

Social aspects

There are very few, if any, aspects of daily living that remain unaffected by the diagnosis of epilepsy. Restrictions on independence can be the most socially disabling – in particular the effects of epilepsy on employment, driving, life insurance and lifestyle.

Employment is important for self-esteem, supporting an independent lifestyle, and affording health insurance and the costs of epilepsy treatment. Numerous surveys show that rates of unemployment and underemployment are much higher in patients with epilepsy than in the general population. Factors most often cited are lack of available transportation (particularly if seizures preclude driving), negative attitudes of employers and employees towards epilepsy, and lack of experience in the workplace. Patients whose education was interrupted by epilepsy-related complications may need additional vocational training before they seek employment.

Clinicians should encourage their patients to work whenever possible and to recommend they seek legal help if they encounter discrimination in the workplace. In the USA, the Americans with Disabilities Act, which was amended in 2008 to further protect the rights of persons with epilepsy, protects a person from being denied employment because of a medical condition if that person can perform the essential duties of that job. In the UK, in line with several other European countries, a similar Disabilities Discrimination Act was introduced in 1995 to protect people with disabilities from discrimination in employment. Whether patients should disclose their epilepsy before being hired is best dealt with on a case-by-case basis.

Driving is often viewed as essential to holding a job and living independently. However, as driving is a privilege, applicants must meet the requirements established by their state, province or country to qualify for a driver's license. With reference to epilepsy, these requirements usually specify a seizure-free interval necessary for driving, the obligations of the patient and the physician to notify the authorities of the patient's status, and allowances that are made under certain circumstances such as seizures that only occur during sleep or seizures that occur during a physician-prescribed AED taper. Clinicians should be thoroughly familiar with the applicable laws where they practice, and should clearly document their discussions with patients. Clinicians should also remember that side effects of AEDs, especially sedation, may interfere with a patient's ability to safely operate a vehicle, and should advise patients accordingly.

Life insurance. Patients with epilepsy may be unable to find affordable life insurance, particularly if applying for an individual policy. Most insurance companies ascribe a globally higher risk of mortality to people with seizures, irrespective of the applicant's frequency or severity of seizures. Patients who obtain life insurance through their place of employment generally do not have a problem.

Lifestyle considerations. Clinicians should counsel patients on lifestyle modifications that reduce the risk of provoking seizures and help maintain overall health without unduly limiting activities that bring enjoyment and fulfillment. Reducing or eliminating the consumption of alcohol, engaging in stress-reducing behaviors, eating regularly and getting adequate sleep may help to reduce seizure frequency. Regular aerobic exercise, especially conducted in such a way that having a seizure would not pose a safety risk, is important for general maintenance of health as well as bone health. Participation in organized sports is generally possible, though the possibility of concussion should be minimized and athletes should consider discussing their condition with team trainers and doctors in advance.

Key points – quality of life

• Depression and anxiety are common in patients with epilepsy, and have a significantly negative impact on quality of life.
• The potential benefit of treating depression and anxiety pharmacologically outweighs the risk of increased seizures.
• Psychosis is uncommon in patients with epilepsy, and generally occurs following a cluster of complex partial seizures.
• When psychotropic medications and antiepileptic drugs are coadministered, dosages may need to be adjusted because of potential pharmacokinetic interactions.
• Patients should be encouraged to work whenever possible, and to seek legal help if they encounter discrimination in the workplace.
• Legal restrictions on driving for people with epilepsy vary; clinicians should be aware of the relevant laws in their place of practice, and must clearly document their discussion with patients.
• Patients with epilepsy may have difficulty in finding affordable life insurance.
• Patients should be counseled on lifestyle modifications that reduce the risk of provoking seizures without unduly limiting activities.

Key references

Arida RM, Scorza FA, Gomes da Silva S et al. The potential role of physical exercise in the treatment of epilepsy. *Epilepsy Behav* 2010;17: 432–5.

Berg AT. Epilepsy, cognition and behaviour: the clinical picture. *Epilepsia* 2011;52(suppl 1):7–12.

Cramer JA, Blum D, Reed M, Fanning K; Epilepsy Impact Project Group. The influence of comorbid depression on quality of life for people with epilepsy. *Epilepsy Behav* 2003;4:515–21.

Fisher RS, Vickrey BG, Gibson P et al. The impact of epilepsy from the patient's perspective I. Descriptions and subjective perceptions. *Epilepsy Res* 2000; 41:39–51.

Gilliam F, Kuzniecky R, Faught E et al. Patient-validated content of epilepsy-specific quality-of-life measurement. *Epilepsia* 1997;38: 233–6.

Kanner AM. Psychosis of epilepsy: a neurologist's perspective. *Epilepsy Behav* 2000;1:219–27.

Kerr MP, Mensah S, Besag F et al. International consensus clinical practice statements for the treatment of neuropsychiatric conditions associated with epilepsy. *Epilepsia* 2011;52:2133–8.

Koch-Stoecker S. Antipsychotic drugs and epilepsy: indications and treatment guidelines. *Epilepsia* 2002;43(suppl 2):19–24.

Kwan P, Yu E, Leung H et al. Association of subjective anxiety, depression and sleep disturbance with quality-of-life ratings in adults with epilepsy. *Epilepsia* 2009;50: 1059–66.

Loring DW, Marino S, Meador KJ. Neuropsychological and behavioural effects of antiepilepsy drugs. *Neuropsychol Rev* 2007;17:413–25.

Noe KH, Locke DE, Sirven JI. Treatment of depression in patients with epilepsy. *Curr Treat Options Neurol* 2011;13:371–9.

Schmitz B. Antidepressant drugs: indications and guidelines for use in epilepsy. *Epilepsia* 2002;43(suppl 2):14–18.

Torta R, Keller R. Behavioral, psychotic, and anxiety disorders in epilepsy: etiology, clinical features, and therapeutic implications. *Epilepsia* 1999;40(suppl 10):S2–20.

A change in approach

With an expanding range of new antiepileptic drugs (AEDs) and anticonvulsive devices that have differing mechanisms of action, there is an imperative to replace the largely empirical approach to the pharmacological management of epilepsy with a more science-based rationale governing choice of therapy. Linked to this must be a better understanding of how seizures are generated and propagated in the brains of individual patients to provide classifications that have a neurobiological rather than an observational basis, ideally with implications for the choice of AED or device. These developments will underpin a patient-centered mechanistic approach to the management of epilepsy. It is, therefore, encouraging that there has been a more focused approach in developing AEDs with novel mechanisms of action that act on molecular targets derived from advances in the knowledge of seizure pathogenesis. Current therapy aims to prevent seizures; future treatments should influence the natural history of the epileptic process. The identification of biomarkers for both disease susceptibility and drug resistance would be a crucial step in achieving this goal.

Genetic progress

Genetic polymorphisms could represent one type of marker. The genes underlying a range of epilepsies are beginning to yield their secrets. With genome-sequencing technologies advancing at a breathtaking pace, there is hope that the genetic basis of the common epilepsies will be unravelled, pointing to new understanding of the pathological pathways and novel therapeutic targets. This approach will contribute substantially to the refinement of the seizure and epilepsy syndrome classifications, and encourage AED development based on pharmacogenomics. Indeed, with the recommendation to perform HLA genotyping before starting carbamazepine in individuals with a high-risk ethnic background (see page 44), pharmacogenomics is

137

beginning to affect clinical practice. The prospect of predicting drug response based on individual genotype offers the possibility of significant health benefits to patients. The challenge remains in integrating pharmacogenetic testing into routine clinical practice.

The introduction of 'gene therapy' for the progressive myoclonic epilepsies and other devastating syndromes is a long-term goal that requires a better understanding of their functional bases.

Pharmacogenomics may also offer other therapeutic opportunities, such as reversal of drug transporter activity within the blood–brain barrier and around lesional epilepsies, which have been implicated in the development of pharmacoresistance. The long-term hope is that the most appropriate AED for an individual patient could be identified with a single straightforward DNA test undertaken at the time of diagnosis.

Surgery and devices

Surgery is considered the treatment of choice for many patients with lesional epilepsies. This must be performed early, before the deleterious effects of repeated seizures produce irreversible neuronal damage, cognitive impairment and psychosocial dysfunction. Epilepsy surgery has been shown to be cost-effective compared with lifelong treatment with one or more of the newer AEDs. Advances in brain imaging are increasingly able to identify patients suitable for surgery early in the course of the disorder and also help to delineate more precisely the target area for resection.

A range of brain stimulation techniques are being devised for patients whose seizures are resistant to AED therapy and who are not suitable for surgery. Electrical stimulation of the anterior nucleus of the thalamus has recently been approved in Europe for this patient population (see page 105). It is likely that this represents the first of many direct brain stimulation devices for the treatment of epilepsy. For instance, with a responsive system, it may soon be possible to increase inhibition or damp down excitation in an epileptic focus by local release of small amounts of a drug or by electrical stimulation in response to burst firing in a coterie of dysfunctioning neurons.

Continued advances

Advances in the understanding, investigation and treatment of epilepsy are continuing apace. Many more people with epilepsy can expect to have their seizures controlled pharmacologically without debilitating side effects. A wider range of medical and surgical strategies are becoming available to optimize treatment for patients with more severe seizure disorders. The development of potentially revolutionary therapies will require close liaison between scientists, bioinformaticians, engineers and clinicians to coordinate theory with implementation, thereby improving the lives of many more people with epilepsy over the next decade.

Useful resources

Evidence-based guidelines
Evidence-based guidelines are increasingly influencing everyday clinical practice. They can be defined as 'systematically developed statements to assist practitioner and patient decisions about appropriate health care for specific clinical circumstances' (Field MJ, Lohr KN. *Clinical Guidelines: Directions for a New Program.* Washington DC: Academy Press, 1990). Guidelines relating to epilepsy and its treatment include:

- www.aan.com/professionals/practice/guideline (American Academy of Neurology)
- www.ilae.org/Visitors/Centre/Guidelines.cfm (International League Against Epilepsy)
- http://guidance.nice.org.uk/CG137 (National Institute for Health and Clinical Excellence, UK)
- www.sign.ac.uk/pdf/sign70.pdf; www.sign.ac.uk/pdf/pat81.pdf (Scottish Intercollegiate Guidelines Network).

Professional organizations
American Academy of
Neurology
Toll-free: 1 800 879 1960
Tel: +1 651 695 2717
www.aan.com

American Epilepsy Society
Tel: +1 860 586 7505
www.aesnet.org

Association of British
Neurologists
Tel: +44 (0)20 7405 4060
info@theabn.org
www.theabn.org

Brainwave
The Irish Epilepsy Association
Tel: +353 (0)1 455 7500
info@epilepsy.ie
www.epilepsy.ie

British Paediatric Neurology
Association
Tel: +44 (0)1204 492888
info@bpna.org.uk
www.bpna.org.uk

International League Against
Epilepsy
Tel: +1 860 586 7547
www.ilae.org

Primary Care Neurology Society
Tel: +44 (0)20 3479 5111
info@p-cns.org.uk
www.p-cns.org.uk

Patient support groups
Epilepsy Action (UK)
UK helpline: 0808 800 5050
Tel: +44 (0)113 210 8850
helpline@epilepsy.org.uk
www.epilepsy.org.uk

Epilepsy.com (USA)
Tel: +1 540 687 8077
info@epilepsytherapyproject.org
www.epilepsy.com
http://professionals.epilepsy.com

Epilepsy Foundation (USA)
Tel: 1 800 332 1000
contactus@efa.org
www.epilepsyfoundation.org

International Bureau for
Epilepsy
Tel: +353 (0)1 210 8850
ibedublin@eircom.net
www.ibe-epilepsy.org

Joint Epilepsy Council of the UK
and Ireland
Tel: +44 (0)1943 871852
www.jointepilepsycouncil.org.uk

Epilepsy Society (UK)
Tel: +44 (0)1494 601300
Helpline: +44 (0)1494 601400
www.epilepsysociety.org.uk

SUDEP, Epilepsy Bereaved (UK)
Tel: +44 (0)1235 772850
Bereavement line:
+44 (0)1235 772852
information@epilepsybereaved.
org.uk
www.sudep.org

Young Epilepsy (UK)
Tel: +44 (0)1342 832243
www.youngepilepsy.org.uk

Index